PSYCHOPHARMACOLOGY

IN

CHILDHOOD

AND

ADOLESCENCE

Psychopharmacology
IN
Childhood
AND
Adolescence

EDITED BY

Jerry M. Wiener, M.D.

BASIC BOOKS, INC., PUBLISHERS

NEW YORK

Library of Congress Cataloging in Publication Data

Main entry under title:
Psychopharmacology in childhood and adolescence.

Includes index.
1. Psychopharmacology. 2. Child psychiatry.
3. Adolescent psychiatry. I. Wiener, Jerry M.
RJ504.7.P79   618.9′28′918   76–43489
ISBN: 0–465–06744–1

DEDICATED TO MY CHILDREN:

Matthew, Ethan, Ross, and Aaron

The Contributors

MAGDA CAMPBELL, M.D., Associate Professor of Psychiatry, New York University School of Medicine, New York, New York.

DENNIS P. CANTWELL, M.D., Assistant Professor of Psychiatry and Director of Residency Training in Child Psychiatry, University of California School of Medicine, Los Angeles, California.

C. KEITH CONNERS, PH.D., Associate Professor of Psychiatry and Program Director of Developmental Neurobiology, University of Pittsburgh School of Medicine, Pittsburgh, Pennsylvania.

MICHELE DANISH, PHARM.D., Clinical Associate, Department of Pediatrics, University of Pennsylvania School of Medicine, Philadelphia, Pennsylvania.

LAWRENCE M. GREENBERG, M.D., Professor of Psychiatry and Director, Division of Child and Adolescent Psychiatry, University of Minnesota School of Medicine, Minneapolis, Minnesota.

STEVEN JAFFE, M.D., Assistant Clinical Professor of Psychiatry (Child Psychiatry), Emory University School of Medicine, Atlanta, Georgia.

REGINALD S. LOURIE, M.D., Emeritus Professor of Child Health and Development and Psychiatry and Behavioral Sciences, George Washington University School of Medicine, Washington, D.C.

ALEXANDER R. LUCAS, M.D., Professor of Psychiatry, Mayo Medical School and Head of Section of Child and Adolescent Psychiatry, Mayo Clinic, Rochester, Minnesota.

JOSEPH H. PATTERSON, M.D., Professor of Pediatrics, Emory University School of Medicine and Pediatrician-in-Chief, Henrietta Egleston Hospital for Children, Woodruff Medical Center, Atlanta, Georgia.

ALBERT W. PRUITT, M.D., Associate Professor of Pediatrics, Emory University School of Medicine, Atlanta, Georgia.

THEODORE SHAPIRO, M.D., Professor of Psychiatry and Director of Child Psychiatry, Department of Psychiatry, Cornell University School of Medicine, and the New York Hospital, New York, New York.

JAMES H. STEPHANS, M.D., Assistant Professor of Psychiatry, University of Minnesota School of Medicine, Minneapolis, Minnesota.

JERRY M. WIENER, M.D., Chairman, Department of Psychiatry, Children's Hospital National Medical Center and Professor of Psychiatry and Behavioral Sciences and Child Health and Development, George Washington University School of Medicine, Washington, D.C.

SUMNER J. YAFFE, M.D., Professor of Pediatrics, University of Pennsylvania School of Medicine and Chief, Division of Clinical Pharmacology, Children's Hospital of Philadelphia, Philadelphia, Pennsylvania.

Contents

Part I

THE BASIC ISSUES

Part II

THE CLINICAL APPLICATIONS

Part III

CONCLUSION AND PROSPECT

Preface

This book came about somewhat serendipitously, or at least inadvertently. Both as a teacher and as a clinician I had experienced recurrent frustration at the absence of an organized source of information in the field of childhood and adolescent psychopharmacology. At the same time I was increasingly interested in the advances in knowledge beginning to occur for understanding the biological aspects of both normal development and childhood psychopathology.

The time seemed overdue for a book on the psychopharmacology of childhood and adolescent disorders. Accordingly, I suggested to several others that they write or edit such a book, but found that all were disinclined at the time to undertake such a project. Each one, however, agreed upon the need, and out of that consensus I myself decided to undertake the book as editor. The job of editor may be compared to the opera conductor's task of orchestrating into a harmonized production the arias from a number of prima donnas (or "primo dons"). The contributors to this book are a group of star performers, and the effort of editing has been stimulating, at times frustrating, but always greatly rewarding.

My supporting cast has been of inestimable assistance, and special appreciation must go to Jean Penn, Sherri Rutledge, Shirley Wells, and Cindy Carroll for their typing of the manuscript, and to my wife Louise for her editorial suggestions and her patience.

PSYCHOPHARMACOLOGY
IN
CHILDHOOD
AND
ADOLESCENCE

INTRODUCTION

Reginald S. Lourie, M.D.

This is a highly appropriate time for a thorough review of the state of the art in the use of the relatively new and proliferating psychopharmacological agents for the organically and psychologically based mental disorders of children and youth. Their availability and the awareness of their usefulness began about forty years ago, which is the biblical timetable for being led out of the wilderness. Particularly in their application for relief of symptoms in the young, mixed messages have been received about such fundamentals as indications and dosage. This book is a scholarly approach to assessing what is known as a sound basis for clarifying guidelines for both the clinician and the investigator.

From the beginnings of recorded history man has used drugs in one form or another to relieve discomfort, elevate feelings, alter moods, stay awake, get to sleep, modify anxiety, and enhance relaxation. This is still true in every culture. In changing societies and even in our inner cities, traditional herb medicines and primitive treatments compete or coexist with more scientific mind-altering pharmacological approaches. When the child was seen as a homunculus, what was good for the adult was good for the child. Even into this century, spirits as a medicine were used to quiet irritable babies. Into the 1930s surgery on infants was not infrequently carried out with the baby sucking on a gauze teat soaked in whiskey and sugar. One must suspect that there is still much that modern pharmacology can learn from investigations of "traditional" medications handed down through the centuries. We must remember that *Rauwolfia* was discovered by scientific studies of an East Indian folk remedy. The blending of the old and new was dramatized by a visit made in the late sixties by Professor Seguin, Chairman of the Department of Psychiatry at the medical school in Lima, Peru, with his residents to observe the chief medicine man in a Peruvian mountain Indian village. Impressed with the medicine man's results from using primitive drug treatment, Professor Seguin asked if he could send his residents to observe further. The medicine man agreed if Professor Seguin would allow the Indian trainees to observe in Lima.

As psychopharmacology came into its own as a scientific field the more casual approach to medicating children made almost a complete turnabout. Until comparatively recently there has been an understandable reluctance to include children in the investigations into the newer psychopharmacological agents. Some of this reluctance can be traced to studies of the action of the then most popular tranquilizer, phenobarbital. In the late 1940s and early 1950s it was found that in the infant and the child under three phenobarbital passed the blood-brain barrier in much smaller amounts than in older children. Therefore, the very young child required nearly adult doses for the drug to be effective. This highlighted the vast unknown area of the relationships between the actions of active nervous system agents and the developing brain at different stages of growth in the young. It is still relatively unexplored. Add to this the problems posed by individual differences as illustrated by the "paradoxical" reaction of the barbiturates in constitutionally hyperactive children. Add further the ethical and moral questions being raised currently about violations of the rights of children involved in research projects and one sees how complex is the process of gaining more information concerning the action of drugs on neural mechanisms in the young. Yet it must be done. Fortunately, some brave and cautious steps are being taken with children at the intramural research program of the National Institute of Mental Health and a few other centers, with investigators working at the cellular and molecular levels in probing drug action and nervous system function.

At the clinical level this uncertainty and lack of clarity about the applications of the newer psychopharmacologicals is reflected in the cautious and therefore often ineffective patterns of their usage with children and adolescents. A survey of pediatricians and family practitioners indicated that while there were many who prescribed them, they did so chiefly in crisis situations, usually in small doses and often on a one-time basis. The exception has been the use of stimulants, particularly methylphenidate and dextroamphetamine, for hyperactive children and those with learning difficulties and the poorly-defined syndrome, minimal brain dysfunction. These drugs have been widely used without adequate diagnosis and/or follow-up and often in response to pressure on physicians by teachers, counselors, and parents. A wave of reaction has taken place with widespread publicity, congressional hearings and the HEW "Daniel Freedman Committee" study and report. Unfortunately misuse continues, although it is decreasing slightly. At the same time these front-line physicians have for the most part given up the older, tried and true medications for children. Chloral hydrate, bromides, paraldehyde, and the barbiturates were and still are useful drugs. All this highlights the timeliness of this book with its summing up and weighing the information and patterns of clinical use of the psychopharmacological agents with balanced, informed recommendations about their clinical application.

It isn't generally known that modern psychopharmacology of children and adolescents has one root which is serendipitous. In the 1930s a pioneer child psychiatrist, Louis Lurie of Cincinnati, explored the relationship of endocrine disturbances to juvenile behavior problems. His only significant finding was that thyroid extract helped hyperactive children to maintain better control. When further explorations eliminated the possibility of hypothyroidism, it became clear that it was the stimulant action of thyroid hormone that was responsible for the calming effect. However, when thyroid extract was used for its new-found sedative effect in the hyperactive, there were a number of predictable side effects when effective dosage was reached. A few others including Langford and Bradley, looking for another stimulant, found that levoamphetamine, then available as Benzedrine, was also effective. Since there were significant side effects, although not as extensive as with thyroid extract, Smith Kline and French was challenged to find another form of amphetamine. Dexedrine was the result.

Another fortuitous finding led to one of the beginnings of the availability of the minor tranquilizers. A new antihistamine, diphenylhydramine, was found by observant clinicians to also have anxiety-relieving and sedative properties. Thus was one of the first of the minor tranquilizers born under the trade name of Atarax. Similarly the antidepressants were developed when it was found that a chemically related drug used in treatment of tuberculosis had mood-elevating effects.

A new dimension has been added to the psychopharmacological scene. In our drug conscious society a significant segment of our adolescent population have become students of drug action. Involved teenagers can quote the literature on the range of "uppers" and "downers" and put many of our professionals to shame. They are representative of an age-old phenomenon, self-medication. Samuel Johnson said that there was something wrong with persons who were not their own doctors by the time they were forty. The precocious awareness of this group of our adolescents would be exemplary if it weren't also used to justify teenage experimentation with drugs. Besides the only too familiar results of drug abuse in this group, the adolescents are being watched by their younger brothers and sisters, who become students of their parents' medicine chests. They should be made aware that we know little about the effects of drugs on their developing nervous systems, even though they may see themselves and act as though they are fully developed.

Dr. Wiener and his prestigious colleagues have carried out a thorough and most useful survey of the state of the art in the still growing field of psychopharmacology in childhood and adolescence. The historical, theoretical, factual, methodological, developmental, and ethical background discussions are authoritative. The section on the use of psychopharmacological agents in specific syndromes should be especially valuable to clinicians because it represents the judgment and experience of many of the most knowledgeable investigators in the child psychiatry field.

Drs. Wiener and Jaffe have made a unique contribution in tracing out the history of drug therapy in child and adolescent disorders. It reflects the growing interest and activity in this area by devoting increasingly expanded historical coverage, decade by decade, from the 1930s to the present day. Yaffe and Danish, as they review the classifications of drugs useful in pediatric psychopharmacology find that without specific data available from replicated research, they must use general pediatric drug experience. They point at the same time to where further work must be done.

Shapiro reviews what is known about a most important area, that of the developmental aspects of use of psychotropic medications in childhood and adolescent behavior "modulating" (as he suggests we call it, rather than seeing it as controlling or otherwise influencing behavior). He builds a bridge to the considerations of such drug use in clinical syndromes when he points out the importance of understanding the nature of the disorder in developmental terms. It is significant from this viewpoint that the chapters on the treatment of childhood and adolescent schizophrenia, the depressive reactions, and special syndromes all review the nature and roots of the specific entities being discussed as the basis for the most enlightened psychopharmacological approach to them. Thus there are available here not only guidelines for drug use, but also a well-informed perspective on what is known about the conditions being reviewed.

The readers of this book must emerge impressed with the repeated admonition that drug treatment never should be seen as curative alone. It is true, for example, that there are children with enuresis (see ch. nine) in whom this symptom continues even after the dynamic and genetic underlying determinants are no longer present. Often these children need a face-saving reason to relinquish the symptom. In such situations not only can the psychopharmacological agents be effective, but also the more than two hundred remedies reported in the literature for this manifestation. However, in the cases reaching the child psychiatrist usually only the more superficial approaches to the problem have been tried. The warning here that should always be kept in mind is that it is essential to pay attention to the basic needs of the patients at the very time that drug treatment has made them more available for such help.

We are grateful to Jerry Wiener and his outstanding colleagues who have shared with us their picture of where we are and where we should be going in utilization of a therapeutic tool with great potential. Freud said, even as he wrote "Anatomy is Destiny," that the ultimate answers to the problems he studied would come from the laboratory. The studies reported here represent a large step in the direction toward which he said he had no time to go himself. The future of this field is in the clinical and basic science laboratories such as those of the workers represented in this volume.

Part I

THE BASIC ISSUES

Chapter One

HISTORY OF DRUG THERAPY

IN CHILDHOOD

AND ADOLESCENT PSYCHIATRIC

DISORDERS

Jerry M. Wiener, M.D. & Steven Jaffe, M.D.

A HISTORICAL OVERVIEW OF CHILDHOOD
PSYCHOPHARMACOLOGY

Introduction

A scientific psychopharmacology for childhood and adolescent disorders essentially did not exist before the 1930s. Reflecting the state of the science at that time, Kanner (1935) commented in the first edition of his textbook: "Pharmacological aids are indicated in demonstrable endocrine disorders, in lues, in the epilepsies, in migraine and other severe headaches, and in a number of other conditions. The indiscriminate use of toxics and sedatives as placebos cannot be discouraged emphatically enough" (p. 133). Progress in the field remained minimal until the latter 1950s, as illustrated by the second edition of Kanner's textbook (1957) which included only two pages of discussion and sixteen references on drug therapy.

During the decades of the 1930s and 1940s the entire emphasis was on the use of Benzedrine sulfate and Dilantin sodium with hyperactive, "brain-damaged," and behavior-disordered children. After the introduction of the "tranquilizers" in the 1950s, the number of studies on the use of drugs for the emotional and behavioral disorders of childhood and adolescence increased, at first slowly, and then dramatically. By 1958, Freedman (1958) listed sixty-three references from the literature, covering fourteen different "tranquilizer" drugs and three "stimulant" drugs. Subsequently Eveloff (1966) published an excellent review of the literature on pharmacology in child psychiatry, citing sixty-six articles for the preceding five-year period. He offered a clinical classification which included the major tranquilizers, minor tranquilizers, stimulants (dextroamphetamine sulfate and methylphenidate) and the antidepressants (MAO inhibitors and tricyclic compounds).

In 1956 the National Institute of Mental Health established the Psychopharmacology Service Center to serve as the focal source of support for research in psychopharmacology, (*Psychopharmacology Bulletin,* 1973). Following a Center-sponsored Conference on Child Research in Psychopharmacology, the first NIMH grant to study childhood pharmacotherapy was awarded in 1958 to Dr. Leon Eisenberg of The Johns Hopkins University. This grant was for the study of two major tranquilizers and meprobamate. A second grant for childhood pharmacotherapy was awarded in 1961, a third grant was not awarded until 1968. Although blame for this minimal support has been placed on the unsophisticated state of methodology in the field (Lipman, 1973), nevertheless, a low level of priority seems to have been assigned to research in childhood pharmacotherapy.

As a measure of both progress and the lack of it, and echoing an observation made twelve years earlier by Freedman (1958), Di Mascio stated in 1971 that, "The majority of these articles [in childhood psychopharmacology] show a marked lack of application of sophisticated research techniques required for the appropriate assessment of a drug's actions . . ." (p. 479). He referred by that time, however, to almost 500 articles in the American literature.

It is indeed true that the majority of studies in childhood pharmacotherapy have serious methodological flaws, including absent or inadequate control groups; nonstandardized dosage schedules; insufficient attention to the placebo effect; absent or inadequate attention to standardized observation techniques, rating scales, and other measurements; poorly defined study groups; and an inadequate basis for diagnostic classification of psychiatric disorders in childhood.

At the same time, significant progress can be noted. A wealth of clinical experience with psychoactive medication has accumulated. Studies published in the past few years have been increasingly sophisticated in their attention to considerations of methodology. The field of childhood psychopharmacology is vigorous and expanding. This chapter will trace the history by decades of this growth and expansion. The first two decades (1930–1950) dealt almost exclusively with the stimulants (and anticonvulsants) in hyperactive and brain-damaged children. The decade of the fifties marked the beginning of the so-called modern era in psychopharmacology with the introduction of the major tranquilizers. During the 1960s the antidepressants and new classes of major tranquilizers were introduced, and there was a revival of studies on the stimulant drugs in the hyperkinetic syndrome. This decade was also marked by an increasing concern for methodology and more refined approaches to diagnostic classification.

The decade of the seventies has so far been marked by increasingly sophisticated verification and comparison studies, an expanding base of knowledge about the biological aspects of normal and deviant child development, and a concomitant interest in the kinetics and mechanisms of action of psychoactive drugs in children.

The 1930s

All psychopharmacological agents for the treatment of behavioral and emotional problems in children were first studied in adult populations. In 1936 a series of studies (Sargant and Blackburn, 1936; Meyerson et al., 1936) described Benzedrine (a combination of the dextro- and levo- forms of amphetamine) as a central nervous system stimulant affecting mood and behavior and possibly increasing intelligence. In the next year, Bradley (1937) reported the effects of Benzedrine on behavior problem children in residential treatment at the Emma Pendleton Bradley Home. This report marked the beginning of a clinical psychopharmacology in children. Because of its historical significance and because most of its results were subsequently confirmed in studies with more sophisticated methodology thirty years later, this first report is presented in some detail. Thirty children, ages five to fourteen years and of normal intelligence, received an average morning dose of 20 mg. of Benzedrine during the middle week of a three-week observation period. Diagnostically, the children varied from "specific educational disabilities, with secondarily disturbed school behavior, to the retiring schizoid child on one hand and the aggressive, egocentric, epileptic child on the other" (p. 578). Effects of Benzedrine were rapid and, in many children, remarkable. Fourteen of the thirty improved "spectacularly" in school performance with increased interest, speed of comprehension, and accuracy. This effect appeared on the first day Benzedrine was given and disappeared on the first day it was discontinued. Eight children demonstrated temporary school improvement, five showed no change in school performance but had an "emotional response," and two had no response at all. Under the category of emotional response, fifteen of the thirty became "subdued," which meant that they became placid, easygoing and had decreased mood swings yielding improvement in social relationships. Seven of the children with the subdued-improved emotional response also demonstrated the "spectacular" increase in school performance. Negative responses included three who cried more easily, two who became more anxious, and one who became more hyperactive, aggressive, and defiant. Side effects were delay in falling asleep, malaise, nausea, and epigastric distress.

Twenty children were given EEG's and over half of these were definitely abnormal. Thus, in a small study using careful clinical observation and each child as his own control, Bradley described remarkable changes in school performance and improvement in emotional response level in about half of the children after administration of Benzedrine. Despite these markedly positive findings, Bradley was cautious as to the use of medication affecting behavior and emotions. He stated, "Any indiscriminate use of Benzedrine to produce symptomatic relief might well mask reactions of etiological significance which should in every case receive adequate attention" (p. 584). This approach is as pertinent now as it was in 1937.

In the same year as Bradley's first report, Molitch et al. (Molitch and Sullivan, 1937; Molitch and Eccles, 1937) studied the effects of Benzedrine on preadolescent and adolescent boys who were committed to the New Jersey State Home for Boys. Using a comparison group that received placebo, but without statistical analysis, they reported greater improvement with the drug on the New Stanford Achievement Test and on verbal intelligence scores. In a third study (Molitch and Poliakoff, 1937) eight of the twenty-two most severe enuretics at the Home improved with placebo, while increasing doses of Benzedrine led to continence in twelve of the remaining fourteen.

Cutts and Jasper (1939), also at the Bradley Home, were the first to describe the reverse effects of phenobarbital in certain behavior-disordered children. Twelve children aged seven to ten who had abnormal EEG's and behavior characterized by hyperactivity, impulsivity, and marked variations in personality unrelated to environmental changes were administered Benzedrine and phenobarbital. Seven improved with Benzedrine, while phenobarbital caused an increase of irritability, impulsivity, destructiveness, and temper tantrums in nine.

The 1940s

Bradley continued to study the effects of Benzedrine at the Bradley Home in Rhode Island, while Bender and her coworkers concomitantly studied the effects of Benzedrine on children hospitalized at Bellevue Hospital in New York. Bradley and his group (Bradley and Bowen, 1940; Bradley and Green, 1940) reported that children administered Benzedrine who showed marked improvement in school performance especially improved in arithmetic, but that Benzedrine did not significantly affect performance on the revised Stanford-Binet scale. They concluded that the improved intellectual performance following Benzedrine administration represented primarily an improved attitude by the subject toward the intellectual task.

Bradley and Bowen (1941) summarized their studies on Benzedrine from the previous three-year period. Administered to 100 children with a variety of behavior disorders, seventy-two improved, of whom fifty-four were "subdued" from a hyperactive labile impulsive state, twelve were stimulated from a previously abnormally underactive or preoccupied condition, and six improved in school performance without other behavioral change. Twenty-one were unaffected, and seven had negative effects described as excessive activity or irritability. These results were related to clinical diagnosis but no definite correlation was found. Bradley commented at that time on the chaos in child psychiatric diagnostic classification.

Bender (1942) reported the effects of Benzedrine on forty hospitalized children who were not otherwise accessible to treatment. Dosages at 10 to 20mg. were administered, and results grouped according to a diagnostic classification. In the psychoneurosis group, which included hysterical, depressed, phobic, obsessive-compulsive, and anxiety states, eight improved and four became more tense and irritable. An immediate and dramatic effect was noted in the "neurotic" or "usual" behavior disorder group in the direction of decreased hyperactivity, increased attention span, improved integration, and more constructive activity. Children with schizophrenia, organic brain disease, or psychopathic personalities either did not respond or worsened. One girl with persistent masturbation and sexual preoccupations responded with relief of "sexual tension." Two of four children with severe reading disabilities had a definite increase in attention span and improved motivation for learning. This was the first report of the effects of stimulant medication on children with a specific learning disability. Bender, like Bradley, put into perspective the possible roles and uses of medication. She commented: "The successful use of this drug in the behavior problems in children depends on a clear understanding of the causes of the child's problems, the proper choice of children to receive the drug, and the use of the drug only as an adjunct to adequate personal psychotherapy, tutoring, and social adjustment" (p. 12).

The 1950s

Stimulants

At the beginning of this decade, Bradley (1950) summarized the results of twelve years of study during which Benzedrine and dextroamphetamine were administered to over 350 children under the age of thirteen years. Of the 275 children who received Benzedrine, 60–75 percent improved with 50–60 percent subdued from a previous hyperactive, impulsive state; 20 percent stimulated from a shy, regressing state; 5 percent improved in school performance with no behavioral changes; and no effect was produced in 15–20 percent. Unfavorable responses occurred in 10–15 percent in which excessive stimulation predominated, and a few were excessively subdued. These results were very similar to Bradley's previous report on 100 children in 1941. The effects of dextroamphetamine were compared with those of Benzedrine in eighty-two children; about a third did better with dextroamphetamine and a third did better with Benzedrine.

Bender and Nichtern summarized their clinical psychopharmacological studies and impressions in 1956. Drugs were given to children with a variety of symptoms. If improvement occurred, this drug was then given to other children with the same symptom complex. At least four to five drugs were used on the ward at the same time, with ward personnel generally being unaware of which drug was given. They reported that neurotic behavior patterns responded best to amphetamines with a majority of children becoming quieter, more cheerful and relaxed with decreased mood swings and relief of tension. In comparing Benzedrine with Dexedrine, they reported that Dexedrine was equally effective in half the dose.

Laufer et al. (1957) defined the hyperkinetic impulse disorder as characterized by hyperactivity, short attention span, impulsivity, low frustration tolerance, poor school work, visual motor problems, writing and reading reversals, and poor handwriting. "Although each of these symptoms or any combination may also have a purely emotional origin, this total symptom complex, at the time of its origin at least, does not seem to be related to any particular psychological precipitant, though it may have concomitant psychological effects and sequelae" (p. 38). Laufer stated that the positive effects of amphetamines on behavior-disordered children, as described by Bradley, were observed primarily in children presenting the hyperkinetic impulse disorder. Thus Laufer, also working at the Bradley Home, set the stage for the later numerous studies of the effects of stimulants on the diagnostic grouping of hyperactive children. He further demonstrated that children with the hyperkinetic impulse disorder had a photo-metrazol threshold significantly lower than did children of comparable age without the syndrome. In addition, thirteen of the children with the hyperkinetic impulse disorder who were administered amphetamines demonstrated a rise in the mean photo-metrazol threshold up to the level previously noted as characteristic for children who were not hyperkinetic. Laufer hypothesized that the hyperkinetic impulse disorder was due to a dysfunction of the diencephalon causing unusual sensitivity to stimuli from both peripheral receptors and viscera.

Methylphenidate (Ritalin) was first synthesized in 1954. Although it was hoped that this drug would be a central nervous stimulant free of the side effects and abuse potential of the amphetamines, double-blind studies in adults did not bear this out. (Fisher and Wilson, 1971). Zimmerman and Burgemeister (1958) reported results in a mixed-age (i.e., four to thirty-three yrs.) outpatient population with a variety of emotional problems. Sixty-five percent of those treated with methylphenidate improved, while sixty percent of a matched group improved with Reserpine. Verbal intelligence retest quotients following six months of treatment with either drug were not significantly affected, but results of the motor test favored the methylphenidate group.

The Tranquilizer Medications

The synthesis of chlorpromazine (R.P 4560, Largactil) in 1950 by Charpentier in France initiated the modern era of psychopharmacology (Dundee, 1954). Because of its sedative and hypothermic effects, the drug's original use was as an adjunct and supplement to anesthesia.

Delay and Deniker (1952) were the first to report on the value of chlorproma-zine in psychiatric patients, and the first clinical report of its use as the sole treat-ment drug for psychiatric conditions appeared in July 1952 (Delay et al.).

The first report on the use of chlorpromazine in children appeared in 1953, describing its value in cases of "psychomotor excitement," with favorable re-sults as long as the medication was maintained (Heuyer et al., 1953).

Lehman and Hanrahan (1954) published the first report in the English litera-ture on the use of chlorpromazine in adult psychiatric patients, concluding that "the drug is of unique value in the symptomatic control of almost any kind of severe excitement" (p. 232).

Several studies were published in 1955 on the use of chlorpromazine in three types of children, the "emotionally disturbed," mentally retarded, and cerebral palsied. Except for one study by Freedman et al. (1955a), all the reports in this first round of experience were essentially impressionistic clinical trials. Silver (1955) reported anecdotally on the use of chlorpromazine for the control of restless behavior and "autonomic imbalance." Gatski (1955) and Flaherty (1955) reported on the use of chlorpromazine for emotionally disturbed boys in residential treatment centers, with dramatic improvement in behavior, trac-tability, and social relatedness. The age range in these latter two studies was from six to fifteen years, dosage ranged from 40 mg. to 1000 mg./day, admin-istration and/or observation were nonblind, and there were no control groups.

Bair and Herold (1955) and Rettig (1955) reported on the use of chlorproma-zine in very heterogeneous populations of behaviorally disturbed, mentally re-tarded children and adolescents. Dosages ranged from 75 mg. to 200 mg./day, with an impressive improvement in behavior reported in both studies. Rettig commented that the greater the ". . . actual brain damage, the less the effec-tiveness of the drug" (p. 194). Neither of these studies included control groups or standardized observations and ratings.

Denhoff and Holden (1955) gave chlorpromazine to children with cerebral palsy. Although the anticipated muscle relaxant effect did not occur, they re-ported an improvement in overall behavior in half of the eighteen children stud-ied, allowing for better rehabilitation and function.

Freedman et al. (1955a) presented the results to that time of a three-year psychopharmacology study on the Children's Service of the Psychiatric Division of Bellevue Hospital in New York City. This was a multi-drug comparison study involving 195 boys between seven and twelve years, selected randomly from admissions to the inpatient service. A well-defined methodology is described, including the use of placebo controls, rating scales, and a single-blind drug administration. Comparing six drugs (Benadryl, Tolserol, Artane, Ambodryl, Thorazine hydrochloride, and Serpasil) with one another, the authors concluded that Benadryl (diphenhydramine) had the best overall effect, particularly in children with the diagnosis of primary behavior disorder displaying anxiety. Chlorpromazine in doses from 30 mg. to 100 mg./day was most beneficial for children with a diagnosis of schizophrenia who were "hyperactive." Artane, Ambodryl, and Serpasil were not superior in effect to placebo.

Contributions during 1956 included papers by Heuyer, Freed and Peifer, Hunt et al., and Miksztal. Freed and Peifer reported the first study on the use of chlorpromazine with outpatient children who were "overactive and emotionally disturbed," having a diagnosis of "primary behavior disorder." Twenty-five children ages seven to fifteen years were treated in doses ranging from 10 to 250 mg./day, including a comparison period on placebo therapy. A decrease in hyperactivity, greater calmness, facilitated learning, and better interpersonal relationships were recorded at a level of "marked improvement" in 70 percent of the cases.

Hunt et al. (1956) reported the most ambitious and carefully controlled study of chlorpromazine use in children to that time. They employed a blind chlorpromazine-placebo crossover study in two groups matched for age and, most importantly, for diagnosis. Diagnostic groups included schizophrenic reactions classified as chronic, "subacute and borderline," and acute; primary behavior disorder; adolescent delinquent behavior; and severely brain-damaged children. Although the number in each group was too small for statistical significance, hyperactivity and social relatedness were consistently improved, with the borderline and acute schizophrenic groups most improved. Side effects were minimal and mild as dosage levels increased to the point of drowsiness and sedation.

Two reports appeared in 1957 (Carter and Maley, Tarjan et al.). The latter reported the use of chlorpromazine in a nonblind, nonrandom, uncontrolled study with 278 defective adults and children (141 at nineteen years old or below) with a subjective conclusion of improvement in 70 percent.

Reviewing the field in 1958, Freedman stated: ". . . one is appalled at the number of drugs recommended and the conflicting claims both as to efficacy and absence of toxicity" (p. 573). He criticized the common shortcomings of faulty methodology, lack of adequate controls, and uncertainty of diagnosis. Freedman listed fourteen "tranquilizer" drugs and three "stimulant" drugs for which there was some report or experience in the literature. The tranquilizers were divided into 1) phenothiazine derivatives, 2) reserpine, 3) diphenylmethane derivatives, and 4) the propanediol derivatives, mephanesin (Tolserol) and meprobamate. The stimulants listed were Benzedrine, Dexedrine, and marsilid. Freedman concluded that chlorpromazine was particularly useful in the treatment of hyperkinetic children, particularly when associated with schizophrenia. Of the other phenothiazine drugs—promazine (Sparine), prochlorperazine (Compazine), perphenazine (Trilafon), triflupromazine (Vesprin), and promethazine (Phenergan)—either there were no published reports of experience with children or only subjectively substantiated or unconfirmed impressions.

Of the diphenylmethane compounds, diphenylhydramine (Benadryl) was reported as particularly helpful and superior to placebo at a statistically significant level in "primary behavior disorders displaying anxiety." This conclusion was based on a preliminary report (Effron et al., 1953) and a later single controlled study (Freedman et al., 1955b). Otherwise, the remainder of this group of compounds—azacyclonol (Frenquel), hydroxyzine (Atarax), benactyzine (Suavitil), captodiamine (Suvren)—were all reported of positive or variable usefulness in the treatment of impulsivity, diffuse anxiety, overactivity, behavior disorders, and brain-injured children. However, none of these drugs had been studied with any adequate methodology up to that time, and no subsequent reports of such studies appeared in the literature. It is of some historical interest that Freedman (1958) cited a study by Bayart, presented at a meeting in July 1956, which reported dramatic improvement in 90 percent of children with tics treated with 30 mg./day of hydroxyzine (Atarax). A published report of this presentation cannot be found, and despite this extremely impressive result with a symptom so often refractory to any treatment, no subsequent reports appeared on the use of hydroxyzine for the treatment of children with tics.

For the propanediol derivatives, Freedman cited his earlier experience with myanesin (Tolserol) (Freedman et al., 1955b), and also reported his impression of meprobamate as useful in children with "organic behavior disorders" characterized by symptoms of hyperactivity, restlessness, distractibility, and short attention span.

Between 1957 and 1961 several articles appeared on the use of meprobamate in children with behavioral and/or emotional disturbance (Litchfield, 1957; Kraft et al., 1959; Zier, 1959; Breger, 1961). By and large these studies included heterogeneous groups of children by age, symptomatology, and diagnosis. Dosage ranged from 50 to 1200 mg./day in the various studies, and methodology ranged from absent to minimally adequate except for the study by Breger, which was methodologically sound and concluded that placebo was as effective as meprobamate for the treatment of childhood enuresis. The other studies reported positive to enthusiastic results for meprobamate in the treatment of everything from petit mal epilepsy to schizophrenia, from enuresis to stuttering, and for various behavioral problems. No further studies of meprobamate in children appeared in the literature to either refute or further validate these results.

The 1960s

The decade of the 1960s is characterized by several developments:

1. An almost quantum leap forward in the study of the stimulants in children with the hyperkinetic syndrome.
2. The introduction into childhood pharmacotherapy of two additional classes of phenothiazine compounds; the piperazines: trifluoperazine (Stelazine ®), fluphenazine (Prolixin ®), perphenazine (Trilafon ®), prochlorperazine (Compazine ®); and the piperidine compound thioridazine (Mellaril ®).
3. The first use in children of two additional categories of major tranquilizing drugs— the thioxanthenes and butyrophenones.
4. Use of the antidepressant drugs—MAO inhibitors and the tricyclic compounds—in various categories of childhood disorders.
5. An increasing concern with the methodology required to yield either reliable or valid results, along with attention to the related issue of adequate diagnostic classification.

Stimulants

Fish (1960a) reported the results of treatment with eighty-five outpatient children under age twelve in whom various medications were used as part of overall treatment programs. Nine of twelve children with school phobia had rapid relief of their sexual and hypochondriacal preoccupations in response to amphetamines.

Knobel (1962) in an uncontrolled study treated 150 children with the hyperactivity syndrome with 20–40 mg./day of methylphenidate (Ritalin) for eight months. He reported that 40 percent showed "good" improvement, 50 percent "moderate" improvement, and 10 percent "no" improvement.

Eisenberg and coworkers, after reporting negative results with tranquilizers (Cytryn et al., 1960), began to study the effects of the stimulants on hyperkinetic children. Eisenberg et al. (1963) first studied the effects of dextroamphetamine on the twenty-one most troublesome male adolescents at a state training school. A double-blind, placebo controlled design was used in three groups matched on the basis of symptom scores from behavioral ratings done by cottage parents, teachers, and peers. The three groups were indistinguishable by the pretreatment ratings. At the end of the seven weeks of treatment, the amphetamine group rated significantly superior to the placebo and control groups. Then Conners and Eisenberg (1963) reported a study of eighty-one disturbed children aged seven to fifteen years in residential care who were randomly assigned to drug and placebo groups. The drug group received 30 to 60 mg./day of methylphenidate over a ten-day period. This was a double-blind, placebo controlled study with symptomatology ratings by house parents and child care workers. A statistically significant improvement occurred in the drug group on total symptom score, a paired association learning test and the Porteus Maze test. These two studies established the short-term efficacy of stimulant medication in reducing hyperactivity, distractibility, and impulsivity.

Except for the grants to Eisenberg's group and to Fish's group, there was a hiatus of funding support between 1961 and 1968 from the Psychopharmacology Service Center of the National Institute of Mental Health. Lipman (1973) described the few grants reviewed and not approved as reflecting the unsophisticated state of methodology in pediatric psychopharmacology. Funding support began again in 1968. Conners was given a personal service contract to develop a reliable and sensitive standardized rating system. The Conners Teacher Rating Scale (Conners, 1969) and the Conners Parent Symptom Questionnaire (Conners, 1970) became standard rating scales in most subsequent studies.

Research on the effects of stimulants in the late 1960s was characterized by improved research design and more emphasis on cognitive functioning. Conners et al. (1967) reported on a double-blind, placebo controlled, crossover design study involving one month of 10 mg./day of Dexedrine and one month of placebo administered to fifth and sixth graders referred by the school because of significant academic and/or school behavior difficulties. Significant improvement occurred by teacher ratings for the active drug group, including a reliable increase on that rating scale factor thought to reflect assertiveness and drive.

Milichap. et al. (1968) reported on a double-blind, placebo controlled crossover design study in which methylphenidate at 1.5 mg./kg. for a three-week period was administered to thirty school-age children of normal I.Q. with hyperactivity and school underachievement. Significant and specific beneficial effects attributable to the drug occurred only on the Draw-A-Man and Frostig figure-ground perception test, while the placebo effect equalled the active drug as measured by the auditory perception test, the Frost visual constancy test, and a spatial-relations perception test. Conners et al. (1969) then reported on a placebo controlled, double-blind randomized study of dextroamphetamine in dosages up to 25 mg./day administered to outpatient children referred for problems in learning. Significant improvement attributable to the drug occurred as measured by the Porteus Maze Test, some visual perception, auditory synthesis, rote learning, and reduction of the hyperkinetic factor on parent symptom ratings.

While the milder side effects, such as anorexia, irritability, insomnia, and abdominal pain had been repeatedly described since 1937, it was not until the late 1960s that toxic psychosis (Ney, 1967) and dyskinesia were reported (Mattson and Calverley, 1968).

Major Tranquilizers:

Fish published two companion papers in 1960 (a and b), which introduced most of the important issues that were to occupy the field of childhood psychopharmacology for the next several years. In these studies the use and comparative effects of Benadryl, chlorpromazine (Thorazine), prochlorperazine (Compazine), trifluoperazine (Stelazine), and perphenazine (Trilafon) were reported in a group of eighty-five children under twelve drawn from a private practice population. These papers reported what were probably the first clinical trials with prochlorperazine, perphenazine, and trifluoperazine in children. The conditions of the studies included a total treatment program, an attempt at more precise diagnostic classification, a definition of average dosage in mg./kg. of body weight, the utilization of a variety of assessment techniques to rate different aspects of ego functioning, and the introduction of a developmental approach which defined age as an important variable in drug effect. Fish provided a good discussion of the philosophy and pragmatics of drug administration in children, as well as a description of qualitative differences in potency among the drugs, related more to differences in overall severity of impairment and type of developmental disturbance than to either diagnosis alone or to isolated symptoms.

In a study already mentioned as supported by the first NIMH grant awarded for childhood pharmacotherapy (*Psychopharmacology Bulletin,* 1973), Cytryn et al. (1960) reported the first effort at a methodologically sound clinical study on outpatient children which compared the efficacy of two major and one minor tranquilizers to placebo in children undergoing psychotherapy. Four diagnostic categories were identified: neurotic, hyperkinetic (both constitutional and secondary to anxiety), defective with behavior disorder, and antisocial. None of the active drugs studied—prochlorperazine, perphenazine (Eisenberg et al, 1961), or meprobamate—was superior to placebo for any of the diagnostic groups.

As the methodology of drug studies improved, earlier enthusiastic reports of efficacy underwent modification. Rosenblum et al. (1960) found no advantage for prochlorperazine (Compazine) over either placebo or no drug in affecting behavior disturbance in a group of borderline retarded children. La Veck et al. (1960) reported the first use of fluphenazine (Prolixin) in a double-blind, placebo controlled study of behaviorally disturbed retarded children, finding no statistically significant advantage for the drug over placebo.

In a study mentioned previously, Fish (1960a) reported a beneficial stimulating effect for trifluoperazine (Stelazine) on withdrawn, hypoactive schizophrenic children. Another study in the same year (Beaudry and Gibson, 1960) proposed that trifluoperazine would provide a calming effect in a hyperactive group and a stimulating effect in a hypoactive group of a population of children hospitalized for "behavior disorders . . . with malignant emotional disturbances." Changes occurred in the direction of the hypothesis.

Clinical reports began to appear in the early 1960s on the use of thioridazine (Mellaril), from the piperidine subclass of phenothiazine compounds. Similar to initial enthusiastic reports in uncontrolled studies with earlier "new" compounds, thioridazine was introduced with claims for significant advantages in efficacy and many fewer side effects than the previously used aliphatic and piperazine subclasses of phenothiazines. Le Vann (1961), for example, reported 90 percent "complete or great improvement" with virtually no side effects in children ranging from institutionalized severely retarded to seriously emotionally disturbed at dosages ranging from 40 to 800 mg./day. In a study of outpatient children, Oettinger and Simonds (1962) reported about equally significant improvement (60.6 percent overall) in groupings of children which included the hyperkinetic behavior syndrome and behavior problems associated with retardation or with seizures. Administration of the drug was by a modified single-blind procedure; no suitable control was defined, and the ratings were largely subjective.

However, the reports of fewer side effects with thioridazine than the aliphatic and piperazine phenothiazines encouraged further studies. Shaw et al. (1963) compared thioridazine with trifluoperazine, trifluopromazine (Vesprin) and fluphenazine (Prolixin) in a well-controlled study, but with a very heterogenous group of emotionally disturbed children. They reported no significant differences in efficacy among these four drugs when compared either by diagnosis or by degree of improvement. Alderton and Hoddinott (1964) reported a statistically significant superiority for thioridazine over placebo in a well-designed study of children with aggressive and hyperactive behavior. Another study with double-blind administration demonstrated superiority for thioridazine over amphetamine and placebo on the hyperactive and disturbed behavior of mentally retarded children, but with no significant effect on cognitive functioning (Alexandris and Lundell, 1968). Two further studies compared thioridazine with the butyrophenone compound, haloperidol (Haldol); one in an inpatient population of "emotionally disturbed retarded children" (Ucer and Kreger, 1969), and another a very heterogeneous population of outpatient children being seen in a mental health clinic (Claghorn, 1972). Both were double-blind comparison studies; the first found a statistically significant advantage in efficacy but significantly greater side effects for haloperidol; the second found no significant difference for efficacy between the two drugs.

In addition, experience with chlorpromazine and various of the piperazine class of phenothiazines continued to accumulate through the 1960s. Garfield et al. (1962) compared chlorpromazine and placebo in a well-controlled, double-blind study on children aged six to thirteen in a university residential treatment program. At doses of 75 to 450 mg./day, chlorpromazine resulted in "depressing" and inhibiting certain behaviors; but in the setting of an active treatment program, actual differences in results between the active drug and placebo were quite small. This study, as much as any, underscored the importance over medication of the total treatment approach, consistent with the results of previous studies of drug effect on children in outpatient psychotherapy (Cytryn et al., 1960; Eisenberg et al., 1961).

In the study mentioned earlier by Shaw et al. (1963), four phenothiazines—trifluoperazine (Stelazine) and fluphenazine (Prolixin) from the piperazine class, trifluopromazine (Vesprin) from the aliphatic class, and thioridazine (Mellaril) from the piperadine class—were all reported effective in relieving symptoms of anxiety, excitability, aggressiveness, and impulsivity in a heterogenous group of children in residential treatment, but no drug was superior to the others. This study also reported reserpine, meprobamate, deanol and benactyzine (Suavitil) as ineffective on the basis of screening trials.

One of the more significant papers in childhood psychopharmacology was published by Fish and Shapiro in 1965. Following up on Fish's earlier work (1960a, 1960b), the authors compared chlorpromazine with diphenylhydramine (Benadryl) and placebo in four groups of young inpatient children. To do so, they introduced a concept of classification according to severity and patterns of impairment and deviation in ego function. Their "types" I and II included severely impaired children with low-level functioning; Types III and IV children were more intact and integrated and of higher I.Q., with behavior disorder and/or paranoid thinking. Sixty percent improved with chlorpromazine, forty-three percent with placebo and none with diphenylhydramine (Benadryl). Clearly chlorpromazine was a potent, active, and effective drug, especially with the more severely impaired children for whom the milieu and placebo were ineffective. Moreover, the classification by severity and type of impairment, along with the methodology used in this study, were introduced in the first of a series of valuable studies on severely disturbed young children from the Children's Psychopharmacology Research Unit of the New York University Medical Center and Bellevue Hospital (Fish et al., 1966; Fish et al., 1969; Campbell et al., 1970; Campbell et al., 1972a; Campbell et al., 1972b; Campbell et al., 1972c).

Fish et al. (1966) next reported their results using trifluoperazine (Stelazine) with severely disturbed inpatient preschool children. Utilizing a carefully matched control group, a placebo comparison, ratings by a "blind" psychiatrist, and doses ranging from 0.11 to 1.60 mg./kg./day (6 to 20 mg./day), they found the drug significantly effective for, and only for, the most severely impaired group of children, in particular those with no language function. Trifluoperazine offered no advantages over placebo for the children with language function and with lesser functional impairment (all the children were diagnosed autistic or schizophrenic). These latter children responded most to the ward treatment program. These findings supported an earlier suggestion that the piperazine phenothiazines with stimulating effects increased the responsiveness of severely impaired children (Fish, 1960b) and underlined the usefulness of the typology classification.

In the mid-1960s, reports began to appear on the effect of the phenothiazines in children with the hyperactivity or minimal brain dysfunction syndrome. Werry and coworkers (Werry et al., 1966; Weiss et al., 1968) compared chlorpromazine (a more sedating phenothiazine) with dextroamphetamine and placebo in groups of children carefully selected for normal I.Q. and free of overt neurological disease, so as to be relatively homogenous for characteristics of the hyperactivity or minimal brain dysfunction syndrome. Their studies showed both chlorpromazine and dextroamphetamine to be superior to placebo to a statistically significant degree in the reduction of hyperactivity and without impairment of cognitive functions. Chlorpromazine was more consistent in its effect, but for that group of children who did benefit from dextroamphetamine, the improvement ". . . seems to be superior to that of chlorpromazine," especially in reduction of distractibility. Jumping ahead somewhat, Greenberg et al. (1972) compared the effects of chlorpromazine, dextroamphetamine, hydroxyzine (Atarax), and placebo in a well-designed study on sixty-one boys with the hyperkinetic syndrome, characterized by hyperactivity, impulsivity, poor attention span, and poor academic performance. Consistent with the previous finding, they found both chlorpromazine and dextroamphetamine significantly better than placebo in effecting the behavior of these children, that hydroxyzine was generally ineffective, and that dextroamphetamine produced either strongly favorable or strongly unfavorable reactions, with fewer of the latter.

The remaining major work on the "tranquilizing" antipsychotic drugs during the 1960s and into the 1970s was with two new classes of compounds: the thioxanthenes, chlorprothixene (Taractan) and thiothixene (Navane), and the butyrophenones, haloperidol (Haldol) and trifluperidol (or triperidol). Both of these new classes were introduced first for use in adults in 1959. According to Di Mascio (Di Mascio and Shader, 1970), the thioxanthenes are characterized by less toxicity but a higher incidence of extrapyramidal side effects than the phenothiazine compounds, to which they are structurally very similar. The butyrophenones have a different chemical structure than the phenothiazines with the advantage of greater potency, calming without sedating, and some stimulant-like activity, but were reported to have the highest potential for inducing extrapyramidal side effects.

An early report on the use of chlorprothixene (Taractan) in children compared it to previous results with thioridazine for symptoms of hyperactivity and habit and conduct disorders (Oettinger, 1962). At an average dose of 2.2 mg./kg./day (range 60–200 mg./day), chlorprothixene compared favorably with thioridazine, having a less sedative and a more stimulating effect, but the ratings were not controlled and there was no comparison to placebo.

The first report on the use of thiothixene (Navane) in children appeared in 1966 (Wolpert et al.) and was followed by two further studies (Wolpert et al., 1967, 1968). The latter studies compared thiothixene with chlorprothixene in twenty matched male inpatients ages nine to thirteen years with a diagnosis of primary behavior disorder. Double-blind ratings of improvement consistently favored thiothixene (Navane).

The first report in the English literature on the use of haloperidol (Haldol) in children (except in the treatment of Gilles de la Tourette Syndrome, reported below) appeared in 1965 (Rogers), describing improvement in destructive, aggressive behavior. Two following studies with groups of children hospitalized for severe behavior disorder without psychosis found haloperidol somewhat but not strikingly superior to placebo in affecting aggressive behavior. (Cunningham et al., 1968; Barker and Fraser, 1968). Le Vann (1969) then reported on the use of haloperidol in 100 children and adolescents, both retarded and nonretarded, with behavioral disturbances within a wide range of diagnoses. This was a noncontrolled, nonblind study which reported striking improvement in hyperactive, assaultive, self-injurious, and other disturbed or disturbing behavior, more so in the nonretarded subjects. Ucer and Kreger (1969) compared haloperidol with thioridazine in mentally retarded children, finding haloperidol significantly superior for control of disturbed behavior but also with a significantly greater incidence of extrapyramidal reactions, ataxia, and agitation. This was a reasonably well-designed study except for the heterogeneity of the study and control groups and the rather low mean daily dosage of thioridazine (53 mg./day), which casts some doubt on the validity of the comparison.

This decade fittingly closed with a report by Fish et al. (1969) on the use of another butyrophenone, trifluperidol (or triperidol).

The Antidepressants

The antidepressant medications (MAO inhibitors and tricyclics) were introduced for use in adults in the late 1950s. The first reports on the effects of antidepressants in children was in 1960, when MacLean reported relief of enuresis by administration of 25 to 50 mg. of imipramine (Tofranil) each evening. Munster et al. (1961), and Salgado et al. (1963) reported similar effects in uncontrolled trials. Tec (1963) described three unusual reactions to imipramine which included an allergic rash, relief of sleepwalking and cessation of chronic headbanging. Poussaint and Ditman (1965) reported the first controlled study of imipramine in enuresis with a crossover design on forty-seven enuretic children. In doses of 25 mg. for children under twelve years, and 50 mg. for those over age twelve, imipramine was markedly superior to placebo, both clinically and statistically, in decreasing the frequency of enuretic nights.

In 1968, placebo controlled, double-blind studies (Bindelglass et al.) with crossover (Shaffer et al.) further demonstrated the significant effect of imipramine in decreasing enuresis.

Reports on the use of antidepressants for the treatment of depression in children and for hyperkinetic children appeared in 1965. Lucas et al. (1965) administered amitriptyline (Elavil) in dosages of 30 to 50 mg./day to ten hospitalized children with mixed diagnoses (including psychosis), whose presenting symptom was depression. A placebo controlled, double-blind, crossover study was done for a twelve-week period, yielding equivocal results.

Rapoport (1965) reported a high improvement rate using imipramine in hyperkinetic children, but this was an uncontrolled study. Krakowski (1965) reported on fifty hyperkinetic children given amitriptyline (Elavil) in doses of 20–75 mg./day in a double-blind, placebo controlled study. The nonresponders to placebo and the initial drug group were given amitriptyline and followed for one month to one year, with a good response reported in 70 percent. In an uncontrolled study of 123 children of mixed diagnoses, Kraft et al. (1966), reported a 60-percent improvement (by phone follow-up) after treatment with amitriptyline. Kurtis (1966) reported improvement in sixteen hospitalized psychotic children who received nortriptyline (Aventil) in an uncontrolled study. In a double-blind, crossover outpatient study of thirty-one patients diagnosed as having depressive illness, Frommer (1967) compared combined phenelzine (an MAO inhibitor) and chlordiazepoxide (Librium) with treatment by phenobarbitone combined with an inert capsule. About half of these patients had phobic symptomatology and the other half had depressed mood disorder. The combination of phenelzine and chlordiazepoxide was superior to placebo to a statistically significant degree. Foster (1967) reported an uncontrolled study of twenty-seven children aged three to eleven with mixed behavioral and anxiety symptoms. Twenty-one had moderate to marked improvement after treatment with nortriptyline.

1970 to the Present

The Stimulants

During the 1970s investigators attended increasingly to methodology (Comly, 1971; Steinberg et al., 1971) and to the major problem of diagnostic discrimination. Fish (1971) described many different kinds of hyperactive children, and stimulants as the drug of choice for only some. She described that those behavior disorders which responded included a predominance of negativism, belligerence, and aggressive behavior. The immature, inadequate, labile diagnostic group, who varied on an almost daily basis from being babyish to being negative and aggressive, did not respond to milieu or placebo, but required an effective medication (Fish, 1975).

Conners (1970a, 1971, 1972), utilizing a profile analysis approach, described seven rather distinct subgroupings of children with the hyperactivity syndrome, correlated with specific drug effects and EEG recordings of visual evoked responses. For example, Group I was characterized by very poor eye-motor coordination and a short attention span. Drugs significantly effected the perceptual-motor factor. The visual evoked response of this group showed a very large hemispheric asymmetry, with left side smaller than right. On the other hand,

Group VI children were low in achievement and rated poorly in classroom conduct. Visual evoked response showed marked hemispheric asymmetry (small left-sided amplitudes), and the drug effect occurred on academic performance, especially spelling and arithmetic. Within the seven subgroupings, different patterns of change in perceptual and cognitive abilities resulted from stimulant treatment. Since the effects of stimulants on cognition and learning will vary with the proportional number of each of these subgroupings in the population of children in the study, previously inconsistent results may be better understood.

Using neurophysiological parameters, Satterfield and coworkers (Satterfield et al., 1974; Satterfield, 1975) identified a subgroup of hyperactive children with low CNS arousal as measured by skin conductance level, evoked cortical response and resting EEG. This subgroup had a greater degree of behavioral disturbance in the classroom and a more predictable positive clinical response to methylphenidate.

While most studies suggested that dosage of stimulants be progressively increased until positive effects occurred, Sprague and Sleator (1973) pointed out that beneficial effects in a specific area at one dosage level may be compromised at a higher dose. In a study of twenty-three hyperactive, learning disabled children, the peak effect of methylphenidate on a learning task of short term memory was at 0.3 mg./kg., while the maximum effect on decreasing seat activity was at 0.7 mg./kg. They also reported that decreased retention of learned material as a result of drug therapy (as reported in earlier studies) had not been supported by subsequent investigations.

Attention to drug-drug interactions in psychopharmacology has only recently become prominent. Methylphenidate has been demonstrated to inhibit certain drug-metabolizing liver enzymes causing a prolongation of the half-life of phenobarbital, dilantin, mysoline, imipramine, and desimipramine, which may elevate therapeutic doses to toxic levels. Children on both dilantin and methylphenidate who developed ataxia due to dilantin toxicity have been reported (Fischer and Wilson, 1971).

Recently Safer et al. (1972) reported the possibility of growth suppression in children on stimulant drugs. The mean yearly weight gain of nine hyperactive children maintained on stimulants for over two years was significantly decreased from that expected. Dextroamphetamine inhibition of weight gain was related to dosage, while methylphenidate under 20 mg./day did not affect weight gain. Eisenberg (1972) related an unpublished study by Zike in which there was no evidence of growth suppression in a group of eighty-three hyperkinetic children treated with stimulant drugs for one to eleven years. Beck et al. (1975) found no effect on physical growth as measured by height in a group of thirty adolescents previously treated with methylphenidate for at least six months.

Pemoline (Cylert), a mild central nervous system stimulant, was synthesized in 1913, studied in adult populations during the late 1950s and 1960s, and only recently used in the treatment of hyperkinetic children. Conners (1972), in a placebo controlled, double-blind study with random assignment, in which pemoline was compared with dextroamphetamine, reported that both drugs were significantly effective on the factors of defiance, inattentiveness, and hyperactivity, but dextroamphetamine was effective within two weeks while pemoline effects were different from placebo only after six weeks.

The Tranquilizer Medications

Efficacy comparison studies among the different classes of antipsychotic or neuroleptic compounds so far dominate this current period of childhood psychopharmacology.

Campbell et al. (1970) compared thiothixene (Navane) to the results obtained in a previous study with trifluperidol (Fish et al., 1969). In a well-matched population of ten preschool autistic-schizophrenic children, the two drugs were not significantly different in effectiveness, but thiothixene had a much greater margin of safety with no side effects observed at therapeutic levels.

Waizer et al. (1972) supported this positive impression of thiothixene efficacy on an outpatient population of eighteen school-age children diagnosed by the Creak criteria as childhood schizophrenics. This group of children was considered highly homogenous for severe to moderate illness. Ratings were by a single blind observer, with a preceding period of placebo. They reported thiothixene to be highly effective and very safe at a mean daily dose of 17 mg./day. Significant improvement over placebo occurred in motor activity, stereotyped behavior, coordination and affect, with little improvement in language function in short-term administration.

In a study measuring both clinical change and neurophysiological correlates, Saletu et al. (1974) compared thiothixene (Navane) with placebo in ten hospitalized boys aged five to fifteen (mean age ten), diagnosed as psychotic with long-standing illness and severe functional impairment. Compared to placebo, thiothixene produced a significant and persistent improvement, beginning in the second week, in areas of motor activity, speech, social relationships, affect and behavior disturbance. In addition, the drug treatment period was correlated with a trend towards normalization of the visual evoked potential recorded by the EEG, as compared to normal controls.

Three further studies of haloperidol compared its effects with those of thioridazine (Claghorn, 1972) and with fluphenazine (Faretra et al., 1970; Engelhart et al., 1973). Methodological problems make the results reported by Claghorn difficult to evaluate. The other two studies found haloperidol and fluphenazine to be significantly and about equally effective in producing improvement in the target symptoms of children diagnosed as schizophrenic. Haloperidol tended to be quicker acting and effective at a mean daily dose of 10.4 mg./day (Engelhardt et al., 1973).

By way of some contrast to the above results comparing a butyrophenone with a piperazine phenothiazine, Campbell et al. (1972a) reported a comparison study of trifluperidol ("prototype of a stimulating neuroleptic") with chlorpromazine (a sedating aliphatic phenothiazine), and placebo. Following the methodology previously established by this research group, fifteen preschool severely disturbed children were studied. Trifluperidol was consistently statistically significantly better than chlorpromazine or placebo in producing improvement in functioning and target symptoms. They found consistent sedative effect and worsening of hyperactivity with chlorpromazine.

The other major use of haloperidol has been in the treatment of Gilles de la Tourette syndrome. The first report of such use was by Seignot (1961). Shapiro et al. (1973) cited an additional ten studies between 1962 and 1970 reporting haloperidol as the most effective treatment for the syndrome. These authors summarized their experience with haloperidol in the treatment of thirty-four cases of the Tourette syndrome with a mean age of onset of seven plus years. They reported strikingly successful results in twenty-one of thirty-four cases on whom there was adequate follow-up. These patients required a median daily dose of 4 mg. with a daily maintenance dose ranging from 1.5 to 44 mg. Treatment was described as difficult and trying, requiring a year or more before dose stabilization was reached at a level between incapacitating side effects and symptom relief.

Antidepressants

The use of tricyclic antidepressants for the treatment of school phobia and the hyperkinetic syndrome has received increased attention. Most recently, a serious side effect related to high doses of imipramine has been reported.

Gittelman-Klein and Klein (1970) reported imipramine, at dosage levels of 100–200 mg./day, significantly superior to placebo in inducing school return and in global therapeutic efficacy.

Campbell et al. (1971) found imipramine to be a poor drug for severely impaired psychotic children; it decreased withdrawal and affective blunting, but increased psychotic speech, behavioral disorganization, and excitement. Winsberg et al. (1972) reported on a double-blind placebo controlled study with crossover on a sample of thirty-two children with hyperactivity and aggressiveness who received 15–30 mg./day of dextroamphetamine for one week and 50 mg. three times a day of imipramine for one week. Both drugs decreased hyperactivity and aggressiveness, but only imipramine improved attention span; 69 percent of the sample responded to imipramine and 44 percent to dextroamphetamine. Waizer et al. (1974) then studied nineteen hyperactive school children administered imipramine in dosages of 100–200 mg./day, followed by four weeks of placebo. The drug produced significant improvement in reduced hyperactivity, defiance, inattentiveness, and increased sociability, while behavior deteriorated during placebo treatment. Rapoport et al. (1971) reported a double-blind, placebo controlled outpatient study on seventy-six hyperactive middle-class grade-school boys in whom imipramine in doses up to 80 mg./day was compared with methylphenidate. Both drugs were superior to placebo, but all rating measurements favored the methylphenidate. Follow-up study of these boys (Quinn and Rapoport, 1975) revealed a higher rate of discontinuance of the imipramine compared to methylphenidate. Both drugs were associated with a decreased rate of expected weight gain, but had no effect on height.

Anorexia and insomnia as side effects of the tricyclic antidepressants were described in the 1960s. More recently increased diastolic blood pressure (Rapoport et al., 1974) and precipitation of seizures (Brown et al., 1973; Petti and Campbell, 1975) have been reported. Of most concern are the very recent reports of cardiac arrhythmias as a side effect of imipramine. Although Martin and Zang (1975) reported no substantial changes on the monthly EKG's of twenty-seven children with enuresis receiving imipramine each evening at a dosage of 25–75 mg. (0.7 mg./kg.), Winsberg et al. (1975) reported seven cases of EKG changes in children seven to ten years of age who were receiving higher doses of imipramine for behavior problems. These children received imipramine three times a day at a 5 mg./kg./day dosage, and three of the seven had a first-degree A-V (atrio-ventricular) block. In response to this study, the FDA (Hayes et al., 1975) ruled that the use of imipramine in children for the treatment of depression and behavior disorders is to be considered investigational. The FDA is to propose specific mg./lb. limits, with a recommendation for regular EKG monitoring when dosage approaches these limits. In their review of the problem, they described one fatality in a child with school phobia from a study in which imipramine was given at a dosage of 14.7 mg./kg./day.

Miscellaneous Studies

1. Pimozide

Pimozide (Orap) was introduced in 1968 as the prototype of a class of antipsychotic compounds acting primarily as a dopamine antagonist. In a pilot single-blind, placebo comparison study (Pangalila-Ratulangi, 1973), pimozide was given to ten children, eight with a diagnosis of schizophrenia. The results were encouraging, particularly in improving affective contact and social behavior. However, only three of the nine children who improved on the drug had a clinical relapse when placebo was substituted, indicating the need for more extended double-blind trials.

2. Triiodothyronine (T-3)

A report by Sherwin et al. (1958) noted improvement in two euthyroid autistic boys after receiving triiodothyronine. Campbell et al. (1972c) administered triiodothyronine (T-3) to an inpatient population of sixteen of euthyroid preschool autistic-schizophrenic children with severe developmental deviations. On a daily dose of 12.5 to 75 mg. of T-3, marked improvement was noted in eleven children, consisting of changes in affect, social responsiveness, language production, and self-initiated activity, with decreases in stereotopy, hyperactivity, distractibility, etc. Blind ratings, using treatment results with dextroamphetamine as the control, indicated statistically significant improvement with T-3 in overall symptomatology.

3. LSD

In two papers published in 1962 and 1963, Bender and coworkers reported on the use of LSD-25 in the treatment of hospitalized severly disturbed children with diagnoses of schizophrenia and autism. Favorable results reported included mood elevations, spontaneous play with adults and other children, improvement in social relatedness, responsiveness to contact and affection, and reduced rhymthmic and whirling behavior. The dosage was 100mg. of LSD-25, with the response lasting over several hours beginning 30 to 40 minutes after ingestion. The drug was given one to three times per week over a six-week period. The methodology and data were not presented.

Simmons et al. (1966), commenting on the methodological limitations of the earlier studies, administered LSD to a pair of four-year, nine-month-old identical male twins using an intrasubject replication design with LSD interspersed with control and placebo observations and objective behavior records. Both twins satisfied the diagnostic criteria for childhood autism. Changes included an increase in social behaviors with better eye-to-face contact and responsiveness to adults, an increase in smiling and laughing behavior indicating a pleasurable affective state, and a decrease in self-stimulation behavior. They found the drug responses to be consistent with those reported by Bender and mentioned unpublished data from a population of eighteen psychotic children to whom LSD was also administered. In this more heterogeneous population, there was a tendency for the autistic-like children to respond as described, while the less retarded schizophrenic children became more withdrawn and disorganized. The effects of the LSD were transient and required continued administration.

Despite these relatively optimistic findings, there are no further reports or follow-up on these studies.

4. Anticonvulsants

Merritt and Putnam (1938) reported on the efficacy of dilantin in the treatment of convulsive disorders. Since that time, reports of its effect on children with emotional or behavioral problems have intermittently occurred. Lindsley and Henry (1942) described that dilantin improved the behavior scores of thirteen behavior problem children, but there was no significant difference in mean scores between dilantin and no drug at the conclusion of the study. Brown and Solomon (1942) administered dilantin for seven weeks to seven behavior-disordered adolescents with grossly abnormal EEG's at a state training school and described improvement in three. Walker and Kirkpatrick (1947) administered dilantin to ten behavior-disordered children with abnormal EEG's and described improvement during the nine- to eighteen-month outpatient follow-up. Pasamanick (1951) reported little positive effect of dilantin on twenty-one hospitalized behavior-disordered children aged six to thirteen with abnormal EEG's. One improved slightly with dilantin, another improved markedly on trimethadione. Gross and Wilson (1964) studied forty-eight hyperactive children with abnormal EEG's who were treated with medication. Dilantin was rarely effective, only one child responded well to a combination of diamox and dilantin. Another child with severe temper tantrums and an EEG with left temporal spikes responded dramatically to celontin. Looker and Conners (1970) reported three cases of children who responded to dilantin following nonresponse to stimulant medication. Because these three children had in common a history of violent temper outbursts, seventeen children ages 5½ to 14½ who had a history of periodic outbursts of violent temper were studied in a nine-week double-blind placebo controlled crossover trial of dilantin. They reported no statistically significant group changes attributable to drug effect, and concluded that diphenylhydantoin was of little clinical benefit in a group of children characterized by severe temper tantrums. All of these children subsequently improved with dextroamphetamine or methylphenidate. Millichap (1973), in a study of twenty-two children with learning and behavior disorders reported a significant elevation of the auditory perception quotient following treatment with diphenylhydantoin in a group of children with paroxysmal dysrhythmias. Wender (1971) reported on four children with periodic rather than continuous MBD symptoms who failed to respond to amphetamines, but responded dramatically to diphenylhydantoin. Thus, individual case reports with marked improvement in response to diphenylhydantoin continue to be reported, despite the fact that controlled studies demonstrating positive effects do not exist.

5. Reserpine

A group of studies appeared in the mid-1950s on the use of reserpine in heterogeneous categories of childhood and adolescent disturbances.

Nicolaus and Kline (1955) reported suggestive but equivocal advantage for reserpine over placebo in two groups of adolescent boys hospitalized with diagnoses of schizophrenia and severe behavior disorders.

Zimmerman and Burgemeister (1955) published a preliminary report on the effect of reserpine in children and adolescents hospitalized for behavior disorders who also had seizures and/or mental retardation. The results suggested improvement in those groups considered psychotic. These same authors (1957) reported a placebo controlled study of reserpine effects in children and adolescents with severe behavior disorders. Seventy-five percent of the reserpine group improved, compared to forty percent of the control group, but with no significant difference between the two groups on measurements of verbal, motor, and social intelligence test ratings.

Talbot (1955) administered reserpine to a group of irritable, hypertonic colicky infants, and reported considerable benefit at dosage levels in the range of .3 mg./day.

Lehman et al. (1957) concluded that reserpine was of some limited usefulness in the treatment of autistic children.

6. Lithium

Large-scale studies in the U.S. demonstrating the efficacy of lithium treatment in adults with affective disorders began in the late 1960s. Studies of lithium treatment in children and adolescents have been infrequent and unconvincing. Van Krevelen and Van Voorst in 1959 (Campbell et al., 1972b, p. 235), reported an adolescent retarded boy with alternating depression and hypomanic states who responded to lithium treatment. Annell (1969 a, b), reported on fifteen patients aged ten to eighteen years with serious emotional disorders of a periodic nature who responded favorably to lithium. Dyson and Barcai (1970) described positive lithium response in two hyperactive depressed boys aged eight and thirteen years who were children of lithium-responding parents with manic-depressive illness.

Controlled studies of lithium on psychotic children were reported in 1972. Gram and Rafaelsen, in a placebo controlled crossover study of eighteen chronically psychotic patients aged eight to twenty-two years, described a statistically positive effect from lithium as judged by parent and teacher rating. Campbell et al. (1972b) reported a study of ten severely disturbed preschool children treated in a controlled crossover design comparing lithium with chlorpromazine. Results revealed that lithium treatment yielded improvement, though not statistically significant, in categories of explosiveness, aggressiveness, hyperactivity, and psychotic speech. Greenhill et al. (1973) reported a three-month modified double-blind trial of lithium alternating with dextroamphetamine or placebo in a study of nine severely hyperactive children who had been unresponsive to other medications. Of the eight who completed the study, six showed no improvement or worsening of symptoms with lithium treatment and two, who had been observed to have affective symptoms, had transient improvement. At present, the use of lithium remains at an investigational level.

7. Comparative Drug Studies

Controlled studies comparing drugs of different classification categories in the same population have been done only during the past few years. In a series of

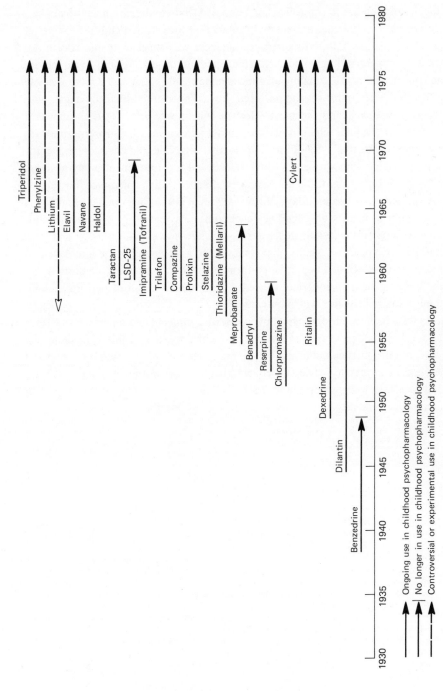

Benzedrine

Dilantin

Dexedrine

Benadryl

Reserpine

Chlorpromazine

Ritalin

Meprobamate

Thioridazine (Mellaril)

Stelazine

Prolixin

Compazine

Trilafon

Imipramine (Tofranil)

LSD-25

Taractan

Cylert

Haldol

Navane

Elavil

Lithium

Phenylzine

Triperidol

1930   1935   1940   1945   1950   1955   1960   1965   1970   1975   1980

 Ongoing use in childhood psychopharmacology

No longer in use in childhood psychopharmacology

Controversial or experimental use in childhood psychopharmacology

TABLE I

double-blind, placebo controlled but uncrossed studies comparing dextroamphetamine, chlorpromazine, and methylphenidate in hyperactive children, Weiss et
al. (1968, 1971) reported that chlorpromazine was superior to placebo in decreasing hyperactivity, while dextroamphetamine decreased both hyperactivity
and distractibility. Dextroamphetamine and methylphenidate had a more variable
effect, but when improvement occurred, it was superior to chlorpromazine, with
methylphenidate being the most effective. Greenberg et al. (1972) compared
dextroamphetamine, chlorpromazine, and hydroxyzine. Chlorpromazine was
moderately effective in modifying hyperactive behavior, and dextroamphetamine
was associated with strongly positive effects and less frequent strongly negative
effects. Chlorpromazine did not adversely affect cognitive and motor functioning
at a dosage up to 125 mg./day. Werry and Oman (1975) in a double-blind crossover study of effects on cognitive functioning in twenty-four hyperactive children, compared methylphenidate at 0.3 mg./kg., haloperidol at 0.25 and 0.05
mg./kg., and placebo. Methylphenidate, and to a lesser extent the lower dose of
haloperidol, facilitated cognitive performance. There was some suggestion that
the higher dose of haloperidol caused a slight deterioration of performance although social behavior was improved.

In this chapter a chronological overview of significant and representative studies on childhood psychopharmacology has been presented. Table 1 illustrates the
years of introduction and/or use for the major pharmacologic agents in child and
adolescent psychiatry. The subsequent chapters, organized by clinical entities
and issues, describe our present understanding and knowledge of this important
therapeutic modality.

References

Alderton, H. R., and Hoddinott, B. A. (1964), A controlled study of the use of thioridazine in the
   treatment of hyperactive and aggressive children in a children's psychiatric hospital. *Canad.
   Psych. J., 9,* 239–247.
Alexandris, A., and Lundell, F. W. (1968), Effect of thioridazine, amphetamine, & placebo on the
   hyperkinetic syndrome and cognitive area in mentally deficient children. *Canad. Med. Assn. J.,
   98,* 92–96.
Annell, Anna-Lisa (1969a), Lithium in the treatment of children and adolescents. *Acta Psychiat.
   Scand. Suppl., 207,* 19–30.
Annell, Anna-Lisa (1969b), Manic-depressive illness in children and effects of treatment with lith-
   ium carbonate. *Acta Paedopsychiat., 36,* 282–301.
Bair, H. V., and Herold, W. (1955), Efficacy of chlorpromazine in hyperactive mentally retarded
   children. *A.M.A. Arch. Neur. & Psych., 74,* 363.
Barker, P., and Fraser, I. A. (1968), A controlled trial of haloperidol in children. *Brit. J. Psych.,
   114,* 855–857.
Beaudry, P., and Gibson, D. (1960), Effect of trifluoperazine on the behavior disorders of children
   with malignant emotional disturbances. *Am. J. Ment. Def., 64,* 823.

Beck, L., Langford, W. S., Mackay, M., and Sum, G. (1975), Childhood chemotherapy and later drug abuse and growth curve: A follow-up study of 30 adolescents. *Am. J. Psychiat.*, *132*, 436–438.

Bender, L., and Cottington, F. (1942), The use of amphetamine sulfate (Benzedrine) in child psychiatry. *Am. J. Psychiat.*, *99*, 116–121.

Bender, L., Faretra, F., and Cobrinik, L. (1963), LSD & UML Treatment of hospitalized disturbed children. *Recent Advances Biol. Psych.*, *5*, 84–92.

Bender, L., Goldschmidt, L., and Siva Shanka, D. V. (1962), Treatment of autistic schizophrenic children with LSD-25 and UML-491. *Recent Advances Biol. Psych.*, *4*, 170–177.

Bender, L., and Nichtern, S. (1956), Chemotherapy in child psychiatry. *New York State J. Med.*, *56*, 2791–2796.

Bindelglass, P. M., Dec, G. H., and Enos, F. A. (1968), Medical and psychosocial factors in enuretic children treated with imipramine hydrochloride. *Am. J. Psychiat.*, *124*, no. 8.

Bradley, C. (1937), The behavior of children receiving Benzedrine. *Am. J. Psychiat.*, *94*, 577–585.

Bradley, C., and Bowen, M. (1940), School performance of children receiving amphetamine (Benzedrine) sulfate. *Am. J. Orthopsychiat.*, *10*, 782–788.

Bradley, C., and Green, E. (1940), Psychometric performance of children receiving amphetamine (Benzedrine) sulfate. *Am. J. Psychiat.*, *97*, 388–394.

Bradley, C., and Bowen, M. (1941), Amphetamine (Benzedrine) therapy of children's behavior disorders. *Am. J. Orthopsychiat.*, *11*, 92–103.

Bradley, C. (1950), Benzedrine and Dexedrine in the treatment of children's behavior disorders, *Pediatrics*, *5*, 24–37.

Breger, E. (1961), Meprobamate in the management of enuresis. *J. Ped.*, Oct. pp. 571–576.

Brown, D., Winsberg, B. G., Bialer, I., and Press, M. (1973), Imipramine therapy and seizures: three children treated for hyperkinetic behavior disorders. *Am. J. Psychiat.*, *130*, 210–212.

Brown, W. T., and Solomon, C. I. (1942), Delinquency and the electroencephalogram. *Am. J. Psychiat.*, *98*, 499–503.

Campbell, M., Fish, B., Shapiro, T., and Floyd, A. (1970), Thiothixene in young disturbed children. *Arch. Gen. Psych.*, *23*, 70–72.

Campbell, M., Fish, B., Shapiro, T., and Floyd, A. (1971), Imipramine in preschool autistic and schizophrenic children. *J. Aut. & Ch. Schiz.*, *3*, 260–282.

Campbell, M., Fish, B., Shapiro, T., and Floyd, A. (1972a), Acute responses of schizophrenic children to a sedative and a "stimulating" neuroleptic: A pharmacologic yardstick. *Curr. Ther. Res.*, *14*, 759.

Campbell, M., Fish, B., Korein, J., Shapiro, T., Collins, P., and Koh, C. (1972b), Lithium and Chlorpromazine: A controlled crossover study of hyperactive severely disturbed young children. *J. of Aut. & Ch. Schiz.*, *2*, 234–263.

Campbell, M., Fish, B., David, R., Shapiro, T., Collins, P., and Koh, C. (1972c), Response to triodothyromine and dextroamphetamine: A study of preschool schizophrenic children. *J. Aut. & Ch. Schiz.*, *2*, 343–358.

Carter, C. H., and Maley, M. C. (1957), Chlorpromazine therapy in children at the Florida Farm Colony, *Am. J. M. Sci.*, *233*, 131.

Claghorn, J. L. (1972), A double-blind comparison of haloperidol (Haldol) and thioridazine (Mellaril) in outpatient children. *Curr. Ther. Res.*, *14*, 785–789.

Comly, H. H. (1971), Cerebral stimulants for children with learning disorders. *J. of Learn. Disabil.*, *4*, 484–490.

Conners, C. K., and Eisenberg, L. (1963), The effect of methylphenidate on symptomatology and learning in disturbed children. *Am. J. Psychiat.*, *120*, 458–463.

Conners, C. K., Eisenberg, L., and Barcai, A. (1967), Effect of dextroamphetamine on children. *Arch. Gen. Psychiat.*, *17*, 478–485.

Conners, C. K. (1969), A teacher rating scale for use in drug studies with children. *Am. J. Psychiat.*, *126*, 884–888.

Conners, C. K., Rothchild, G., Eisenberg, L., Schwartz, L. S., and Robinson, E. (1969), Dextroamphetamine sulfate in children with learning disorders. *Arch. Gen Psychiat.*, *21*, 182–190.

Conners, C. K. (1970a), Stimulant drugs and cortical evoked responses in learning and behavior disorders in children. [In W. L. Smith (Ed.), *Drugs, Development and Cerebral Function*. Springfield: Charles C. Thomas.

Conners, C. K. (1970b), Symptom patterns in hyperkinetic neurotic and normal children. *Child Dev.*, *41*, 667–682.

Conners, C. K. (1971), Recent drug studies with hyperkinetic children. *J. Learn. Disabil., 4,* 478–483.

Conners, C. K. (1972), Psychological effects of stimulant drugs in children with minimal brain dysfunction. *Pediatrics, 49,* 702–708.

Cunningham, M. A., Pillai, V., and Rogers, W. J. B. (1968), Haloperidol in the treatment of children with severe behavior disorders. *Brit. J. Psych., 114,* 845–854.

Cutts, K. K., and Jasper, H. H. (1939), Effect of benzedrine sulfate and phenobarbital on behavior problem children with abnormal electroencelphalograms. *Arch. Neurol. & Psychiat., 41,* 1138–1145.

Cytryn, L., Gilbert, A., & Eisenberg, L. (1960), The effectiveness of tranquilizing drugs plus supportive psychotherapy in treating behavior disorders of children: A double-blind study of eighty outpatients. *Am. J. Orthopsychiat., 30,* 113–129.

Delay, J., and Deniker, P. (1952), Réactions biologiques observées au cours du traitement par le chlorhydrate de diméthylaninopropyl-N-chorophénothiazine (4560 r. p.), Congrès des psychiatres de langue française., Luxembourg, July 22–26.

Delay, J., Deniker, P., and Harl, J. M. (1952), Traitement des états d'excitation et d'agitation par une méthode medicamenteuse derivée de l'hibernotherapie. *Ann. Méd.-Psychol., 110,* 267–273.

Denhoff, E., and Holden, R. H. (1955), The effectiveness of chlorpromazine (Thorazine) with cerebral palsied children. *J. Ped., 47,* 328–332.

Di Mascio, A. (1970), Classification and overview of psychotropic drugs. In *Clinical handbook of psychopharmacology.* A. Di Mascio, and R. I. Shader (Eds.), New York: Aronson, pp. 3–15.

Di Mascio, A. (1971), Psychopharmacology in Children. In *Ann. Progress in Ch. Psychiat. and Ch. Dev.,* S. Chess, and A. Thomas (Eds.), New York: Brunner/Mazel, pp. 479–491.

Dundee, J. W. (1954), A review of chlorpromazine hydrochloride. *Brit. J. of Anaesthesia, 26,* 357–379.

Dyson, W. L., and Barcai, A. (1970), Treatment of children of lithium-responding parents. *Curr. Ther. Res. 12,* 286–290.

Effron, A. S., and Freedman, A. M. (1953), The treatment of behavior disorders in children with Benadryl, A preliminary report. *J. Ped., 42,* 261.

Eisenberg, L., Gilbert, A., Cytryn, L., and Molling, P. A. (1961), The effectiveness of psychotherapy alone and in conjunction with perphenazine or placebo in the treatment of neurotic and hyperkinetic children. *Am. J. Psych., 117,* 1088–1093.

Eisenberg, L., Lackman R., Molling, P. A., Lockner, A., Mizelle, J. D., and Conners, C. K. (1963), A psychopharmacologic experiment in a training school for delinquent boys: methods, problems, findings. *J. Orthopsychiat., 33,* 431–447.

Eisenberg, L. (1972), The hyperkinetic child and stimulant drugs. *N. Eng. J. Med., 287,* 249–250.

Engelhardt, D. M., Polizos, P., Waizer, J., and Hoffman, S. P. (1973), A double-blind comparison of fluphenazine and haloperidol in outpatient schizophrenic children. *J. Aut. & Ch. Schiz., 3,* 128–237.

Eveloff, H. H. (1966), Psychopharmacologic agents in child psychiatry. *Arch. Gen. Psych., 14,* 472–481.

Faretra, G., Dooher, L., and Dowling, J. (1970), Comparison of haloperidol and fluphenazine in disturbed children. *Am. J. Psych., 126,* 1670–1673.

Fish, B. (1960a), Drug therapy in child psychiatry: Psychological aspects. *Compr. Psych., 1,* 55–61.

Fish, B. (1960b), Drug therapy in child psychiatry: Pharmacological aspects. *Compr. Psych., 1,* 212–227.

Fish, B., and Shapiro, T. (1965), A typology of children's psychiatric disorders. I. Its application to a controlled evaluation of treatment. *J. Am. Acad. Ch. Psych., 4,* 32–52.

Fish, B. (1971), The one child, one drug myth of stimulants in hyperkinesis. *Arch. Gen. Psychiat., 25,* 193–209.

Fish, B. (1975), Stimulant Drug treatment of hyperactive children. In D. Cantwell (Ed.), *The Hyperactive Child.* New York: Spectrum Publications, Inc., pp. 109–127.

Fish, B., Campbell, M., Shapiro, T., and Floyd, A. (1969), Comparison of trifluperidol, trifluoperazine, and chlorpromazine in preschool, schizophrenic children: The value of less sedative antipsychotic agents. *Curr. Ther. Res., 11,* 589–595.

Fish, B., Shapiro, T., and Campbell, M. (1966), Long term prognosis and the response of schizophrenic children to drug therapy: A controlled study of trifluoperizine. *Am. J. Psych., 123,* 32–39.

Fisher, K. C., and Wilson, W. P. (1971), Methylphenidate and the hyperkinetic state. *Dis. Nerv. Sys.,* pp. 695–698.

Flaherty, J. A. (1955), Effect of chlorpromazine medication on children with severe emotional disturbance. *Del. St. Med. J.*, pp. 180–184.

Foster, P. (1967), Treatment of childhood depression. *Newton Wellsley Med. Bull.*, *19*, 33–36.

Freed, H., and Peifer, C. A. (1956), Treatment of hyperkinetic emotionally disturbed children with prolonged administration of chlorpromazine. *Am. J. Psych.*, *113*, 22–26.

Freedman, A. M., Effron, A. S., and Bender, L. (1955a), Pharmacotherapy in children with psychiatric illness. *J. Nerv. & Ment. Dis.*, *122*, 479–486.

Freedman, A. M., Kremer, M. W., Robertiello, R. C., and Effron, A. S. (1955b), The treatment of behavior disorders in children with tolserol. *J. Ped.*, *47*, 369–372.

Freedman, A.M. (1958) Drug therapy in behavior disorders. *Ped. Cl. N. Am.*, *5*, 573–94.

Frommer, E. A. (1967), Treatment of childhood depression with antidepressant drugs. *Brit. Med. J.*, *1*, 729–732.

Garfield, S. L., Helper, M. M., Wilcott, R. C., and Murrly, R. (1962), Effects of chlorpromiazine on behavior in emotionally disturbed children. *J. Nerv. Ment. Dis.*, *135*, 147–154.

Gatski, R. L. (1955), Chlorpromazine in the treatment of emotionally maladjusted children. *J.A.M.A.*, *157*, 1298–1300.

Gittelman-Klein, R., & Klein, D. F. (1970) Controlled imipramine treatment of school phobia. *Arch. Gen. Psychiat.*, *25*, 204–207.

Gram, L. F., & Rafaelsen, O. J. (1972), Lithium treatment of psychotic children and adolescents. *Acta. Psychiat. Scand.*, *48*(*3*), 253–260.

Greenberg, L. M., Deens, M. A., and McMahon, A. (1972), Effects of dextroamphetamine, chlorpromazine, & hydroxyzine on behavior and performance in hyperactive children. *Am. J. Psych.*, *129*, 532–539.

Greenhill, L. L., Rieder, R. O., Wender, P. H., Bucksbaum, M., and Zahn, T. P. (1973) Lithium carbonate in the treatment of hyperactive children. *Arch. Gen. Psychiat.*, *28*, 636–640.

Gross, M. D., and Wilson, W. C. (1964), Behavior disorders of children with cerebral dysrhythmias. *Arch. Gen. Psychiat.*, *11*, 610–619.

Hayes, T. A., Panitch, M. L., and Barker, E. (1975), Imipramine dosage in children: A comment on imipramine and electrocardiographic abnormalities in hyperactive children. *Am. J. Psychiat.*, *132*, 546–547.

Heuyer, G., Gerard, G., and Galibert, J. (1953), Traitement de l'excitation psychometrics chez l'enfant paré (le456 r.p.) *Arch. Franc. Pediat.*, *9*, 961.

Heuyer, G., Dell, C., and Prinquet, G. (1956), Emploi de la chlorpromazine en neuro-psychiatric infantile. *Encéphale*, *45*, 576–578.

Hunt, B. R., Frank, T., and Krush, T. P. (1956), Chlorpromazine in the treatment of severe emotional disorders of childhood. *A.M.A. J. Dis. Children.*, *9*, 268–277.

Hunter, H., and Stephenson, G. M. (1963), Chlorpromazine and trifluoperazine in the treatment of behavioral abnormalities in the severely subnormal child. *Am. J. Psych.*, *109*, 411–417.

Kanner, L. (1935), *Child Psychiatry*. Springfield: Charles C. Thomas, p. 133.

Kanner, L. (1957), *Child Psychiatry*. Springfield: Charles C. Thomas.

Knobel, M. (1962), Psychopharmacology for the hyperkinetic child. *Arch. Gen. Psychiat.*, *6*, 30–34.

Kraft, I. A., Marcus, I. M., Wilson, W., Swander, D. V., Rumage, N. W., and Schulhoffer, E. (1959), Methodological problems in studying the effect of tranquilizers in children with specific reference to meprobamate. *South. Med. J.*, *52*, 179–185.

Kraft, I. A., Ardali, C., Duffy, J., Hart, J., and Pearce, P. R. (1966), Use of amitryptyline in childhood behavior disturbances. *Int. J. Neuropsychiat.*, *2*, 611–614.

Krakowski, A. J. (1965), Amitryptyline in treatment of hyperkinetic children: A double-blind study. *Psychosom.*, *6*, 355–360.

Kurtis, L. B. (1966), Clinical study of the response to nortriptyline on autistic children. *Int. J. Neuropsychiat.*, *2*, 298–301.

Laufer, M., Denhoff, E., and Solomons, G. (1957), Hyperkinetic impulse disorder in children's behavior problems. *Psychosom. Med.*, *19*, 38:49.

La Veck, G. D., De La Crug, F., and Simundson, E. (1960), Fluphenazine in the treatment of mentally retarded children with behavior disorders. *Dis. of Nerv. Sys.*, pp. 82–85.

Lehmann, H. E., and Hanrahan, G. E. (1954), Chlorpromazine, new inhibiting agent for psychomotor excitement and manic states. *Arch. of Psych. & Neur.*, *71*, 227–237.

Le Vann, L. J. (1961), Thioridazine, a psychosedative virtually free of side-effects. *Alberta Med. Bull.*

Le Vann, L. J. (1969), Haloperidol in the treatment of behavioral disorders in children and adoles-
    cents. *Canad. Psychiat. Assn. J., 14,* 217–220.
Lindsley, D. B., and Henry, C. E. (1942), The effects of drugs on behavior and the electroen-
    cephalograms of children with behavior disorders. *Psychosom. Med., 4,* 140–149.
Lipman, R. S. (1973), NIMH-PRB support of research in minimal brain dysfunction and other
    disorders of childhood. *Psychopharm. Bull.* Special Issue, Pharmacotherapy of children. NIMH,
    pp. 1–8. DHEW Publication No. (HSM) 73-9002.
Litchfield, H. R. (1957), Clinical evaluation of meprobamate in disturbed and prepsychotic children.
    Ann. NY Acad. Sci., 67, 828–832.
Looker, A., and Conners, C. K. (1970), Diphenylhydantoin in children with severe temper tantrums.
    Arch. Gen. Psychiat., 23, 80–89.
Lucas, A. P., Lockett, H. J., and Grimm, F. (1965), Amitriptyline in childhood depression. *Dis.
    Nerv. Sys., 28,* 105–113.
MacLean, R. E. G. (1960), Imipramine hydrochloride (Tofranil) and enuresis. *Am. J. Psychiat.,
    117,* 551.
Martin, G. I., and Zang, P. J. (1975), Electrocardiographic monitoring of enuretic children receiving
    therapeutic doses of imipramine. *Am. J. Psychiat., 132,* 540–541.
Mattson, R. H., and Calverlez, J. R. (1968), Dextroamphetamine sulfate induced dyskinesias,
    J.A.M.A., 205, 400–402.
Merritt, H. H., and Putnam, T. J. (1938), Sodium diphenylhydantoinate in treatment of convulsive
    disorders. *J.A.M.A., 111,* 1068–1073.
Meyerson, A. (1936), Effect of benzedrine sulfate on mood and fatigue in normal and neurotic per-
    sons. *Arch. Neurol. Psychiat., 36,* 816–822.
Meyerson, A., Lomar, J., and Dameshek, W. (1936), Physiological effects of Benzedrine and its
    relationship to other drugs affecting the autonomic nervous system. *Am. J. Med. Sci., 192,*
    560–574.
Miksztal, M. W. (1956), Chlorpromazine (Thorazine) and reserpine in residential treatment of
    neuropsychiatric disorders in children. *J. Nerv. & Ment. Dis., 123,* 477–479.
Millichap, J. G., Aymat, F., Sturgis, L. H., Larsen, K. W., and Egan, R. A. (1968), Hyperkinetic
    behavior and learning disorders III. Battery of neuropsychological tests in controlled trial of
    methylphenidate. *Am. J. Dis. Ch., 116,* 235–244.
Millichap, J. G. (1973), Drugs in management of minimal brain dysfunction. *Ann. N.Y. Acad. Sci.,
    205,* 321–334.
Molitch, M., and Eccles, A. K. (1937), The effect of benzedrine sulfate on the intelligence scores of
    children. *Am. J. Psychiat., 94,* 587–590.
Molitch, M., and Poliakoff, S. (1937), The effect of benzedrine sulfate on enuresis. *Arch. Ped., 54,*
    499–501.
Molitch, M., and Sullivan, J. P. (1937), The effect of benzedrine sulfate on children taking the new
    Stanford Achievement Test. *Am. J. Orthopsychiat., 7,* 519–522.
Munster, A. J., Stanley, A. M., and Saunders, J. C. (1961), Imipramine (Tofranil) in the treatment
    of enuresis. *Am. J. Psychiat., 118,* 76–77.
Ney, P. G. (1967), Psychosis in a child associated with amphetamine administration. *Canad. Med.
    Assn. J., 97,* 1026–1029.
Nicolaus, P., and Kline, N. S. (1955), Reserpine in the treatment of disturbed adolescents. *Psychiat.
    Res.,* pp. 122–132.
Oettinger, L. Jr. (1962), Chlorprothixene in the management of problem children. *Dis. Nerv. Sys.,*
    Oct., pp. 568–571.
Oettinger, L., and Simonds, R. (1962), The use of thioridazine in the office management of chil-
    dren's behavior disorders. *Med. Times., 90,* 596–604.
Pangalila-Ratulangi, E. A. (1973), Pilot Evaluation of Orap® (Pimozide, R6238) in child psychiatry.
    Psychiatria, Neurologia, Neurochirurgia, 76, 17–27.
Pasamanick, B. (1951), Anticonvulsant drug therapy of behavior problem children with abnormal
    electroencephalograms. *Arch. Neurol. Psychiat., 65,* 752–766.
Petti, T. A., and Campbell, M. (1975), Imipramine and seizures. *Am. J. Psychiat., 132,* 538–540.
Poussaint, A. F., and Ditman, K. S. (1965), A controlled study of imipramine (Tofranil) in the treat-
    ment of childhood enuresis. *J. Ped., 67,* 283–290.
Psychopharmacology Bulletin (1973), Special Issue, Pharmacotherapy of children. NIMH, DHEW
    publication No. (HSM) 73-9002.

Quinn, P., and Rapoport, J. L. (1975), One year followup of hyperactive boys treated with imipramine or methylphenidate. *Am. J. Psychiat., 132,* 241–245.

Rapoport, J. (1965), Childhood behavior and learning problems treated with imipramine. *Int. Jr. Neuropsychiat., 1,* 635–642.

Rapoport, J. L., Quinn, P. O., Bradbard, G., Riddle, D., and Brooks, E. (1974), Imipramine and methylphenidate treatments of hyperactive boys. *Arch. Gen. Psychiat., 30,* 789–793.

Rettig, J. H. (1955), Chlorpromazine for the control of psychomotor excitement in the mentally deficient. *J. Nerv. & Ment. Dis., 122,* 190.

Rogers, W. J. B. (1965), Use of haloperidol in children's psychiatric disorders. *Clin. Trials J., 2,* 162–164.

Rosenblum, S., Buoniconto, P., and Graham, B. D. (1960), ''Compazine'' vs. placebo: A controlled study with educable, emotionally disturbed children. *Am. J. Ment. Def., 64,* 713.

Safer, D., Allen, R., and Barr, E. (1972), Depression of growth in hyperactive children on stimulant drugs. *N. Eng. J. Med., 287,* 217–220.

Saletu, B., Simeon, J., Saletu, M., Itil, T.M., and DaSilva, J. (1974). Behavioral & visual evoked potential investigations during trihexyphenidyl and thiothixene treatment in psychotic boys. *Biol. Psych., 8,* 177–189.

Salgado, M. A., and Kierdel-Vegas, O. (1963). Treatment of enuresis with imipramine. *Am. J. Psychiat., 119,* 990.

Sargant, W., and Blackburn, J. M. (1936). The effect of Benzedrine on intelligence scores. *Lancet,* Dec. 12, pp. 1385–1387.

Satterfield, J. H., Cantwell, D. P., and Satterfield, B. T. (1974). Pathophysiology of the hyperactive child syndrome. *Arch. Gen. Psychiat., 21,* 839–844.

Satterfield, J. H. (1975). Neurophysiologic studies with hyperkinetic children. D. P. Cantwell (Ed.), *The Hyperactive Child.* New York: Spectrum Publications, Inc., 1975.

Seignot, J. J. N. (1961). A case of the syndrome of tics of Gilles de la Tourette controlled by R1625. *Ann. Med. Psych.,* 1961, *119,* 578–579.

Shaffer, D., Costello, A. J., and Hill, I.D. (1968). Control of enuresis with imipramine. *Arch. Dis. Ch., 43,* 665–671.

Shapiro, A. K., Shapiro, E., and Wayne, H. (1973). Treatment of Tourette's syndrome. *Arch. Gen. Psych., 28,* 92–97.

Shaw, C. R., Lockett, H. J., Lucas, A. R., Lamontagne, C. H., and Crimm, F. (1963). Tranquilizer drugs in the treatment of emotionally disturbed children: I. Inpatients in a residential treatment center. *J. Am. Acad. Ch. Psych., 2,* 725–742.

Sherwin, A. C., Flach, F. F., and Stokes, P. E. (1958). Treatment of psychoses in early childhood with triiodothyronine. *Am. J. Psych., 115,* 166–167.

Silver, A. A. (1955). Management of children with schizophrenia. *Am. J. Psychoth., 9,* 196.

Simmons, J. Q. III, Leiken, S. J., Lovaas, O.I., Schaeffer, B., and Perloff, B. (1966). Modification of autistic behavior with LSD-25. *Am. J. Psych., 122,* 1201–1211.

Sprague, R. L., and Sleator, E.K. (1973). Effects of psychopharmacologic agents on learning disorders. *Ped. Cl. N. Am., 20,* 719–735.

Steinberg, G. C., Troshivsky, C., and Steinberg, H. R. (1971). Dextroamphetamine responsive behavior disorders in school children. *Am. J. Psychiat., 128,* 66–71.

Talbot, M. W., Jr. (1955). The use of reserpine in irritable and hypertonic infants. *Ann. N.Y. Acad. Sci., 61,* 188–197.

Tarjan, G., Lowery, V. E., and Wright, S. W. (1957). Use of chlorpromazine in two hundred seventy-eight mentally deficient patients. *Am. J. Dis. Ch., 94,* 294–300.

Tec, Leon (1963). Unexpected effects in children treated with imipramine. *Am. J. Psychiat., 119,* 603.

Ucer, E., and Kreger, K. C. (1969). A Double-blind study comparing haloperidol & thioridazine in emotionally disturbed, mentally retarded children. *Curr. Ther. Res., 11,* 278–283.

Waizer, J., Polizos, P., Hoffman, S. P., Engelhardt, D. M., and Margolis, R. A. (1972). A single-blind evaluation of thiothixene with outpatient schizophrenic children. *J. Aut. & Ch. Schiz., 2,* 378–386.

Waizer, J., Hoffman, S. P., Polizos, P., and Engelhardt, D. M. (1974). Outpatient treatment of hyperactive school children with imipramine. *Am. J. Psychiat. 131,* 587–591.

Walker, C. F., and Kirkpatrick, B. B. (1947). Dilantin treatment for behavior problem children with abnormal electroencephalograms. *Am. J. Psychiat., 103,* 484–492.

Weise, C. C., O'Reilly, P. P., and Hesbacher, P. (1972). Perphenazine-amitriptyline in neurotic underachieving students: A controlled study. *Dis. Nerv. Sys.*, pp. 318–325.

Weiss, G., Werry, J., Minde, K., Douglas, V., and Sykes, D. (1968). Studies on the hyperactive child V: The effects of dextroamphetamine & chlorpromazine on behavior and intellectual functioning. *J. Ch. Psych. & Psychiat.*, *9*, 145–156.

Weiss, G., Minde, K., Douglas, V., Werry, J., and Sykes, D. (1971). Comparison of the effects of chlorpromazine, dextroamphetamine and methylphenidate on behavior and intellectual functioning of hyperactive children. *Canad. Med. Assn. J.*, *104(1)*, 20–25.

Wender, Paul (1971). *Minimal brain dysfunction in children*. New York: John Wiley & Sons, Inc.

Werry, J. S., Weiss, G., Douglas, V., and Martin, J. (1966). Studies on the hyperactive child III: The effect of chlorpromazine upon behavior & learning ability. *J. Am. Acad. Ch. Psych.*, *5*, 292–312.

Werry, J. S., and Aman, M. G. (1975). Methylphenidate and haloperidol in children. *Arch. Gen. Psychiat.*, *32*, 790–795.

Winkelman, N. W., Jr. (1954). Chlorpromazine in the treatment of neuropsychiatric disorders. *J.A.M.A.*, *155*, 18.

Winsberg, B. G., Beater, I., Kupietz, S., and Tobias, J. (1972) Effects of imipramine and dextroamphetamine on behavior of neuropsychiatrically impaired children. *Am. J. Psychiat.*, *128*, 1425–1431.

Winsberg, B. G., Goldstein, S., Yepes, L. E., and Perel, J. M. (1975). Imipramine and electrocardiographic abnormalities in hyperactive children. *Am. J. Psychiat.*, *132*, 542–545.

Wolpert, A., Hagamen, M. B., and Merlis, S. (1966). A pilot study of thiothixene in childhood schizophrenia. *Curr. Ther. Res.*, *8*, 617–620.

Wolpert, A., Hagamen, M. B., and Merlis, S. (1967). A comparative study of thiothixene and trifluoperazine in childhood schizophrenia. *Curr. Ther. Res.*, *9*, 482–485.

Wolpert, A., Quintos, A., White, L., and Merlis, S. (1968). Thiothixene & chlorprothixene in behavior disorders. *Curr. Ther. Res.*, *10*, 566–569.

Zier, A. (1959). Meprobamate (Miltown) as an Aid to Psychotherapy in an Outpatient Child Guidance Clinic. *Am. J. Ortho.*, *29*, 377–382.

Zimmerman, F. T., and Burgemeister, B. (1955). Preliminary report upon the effect of reserpine upon epilepsy and behavior problems in children. *Ann. N.Y. Acad. Sci.*, *61*, 215–221.

Zimmerman, F. T., and Burgemeister, B. B. (1957). The effect of reserpine on the behavior problems of children. *N.Y. St. J. Med.*, pp. 3132–3140.

Zimmerman, F. T., and Burgemeister, B. B. (1958), Action of methyl-phenidate (Ritalin) and reserpine in behavior disorders in children and adults. *Am. J. Psychiat.*, *115*, 323–328.

Chapter Two

THE CLASSIFICATION AND PHARMACOLOGY OF PSYCHOACTIVE DRUGS IN CHILDHOOD AND ADOLESCENCE

Sumner J. Yaffe, M.D. & Michele Danish, PHARM.D.

INTRODUCTION

The classification of psychotropic or psychoactive agents for use in children and adolescents is greatly hampered by the lack of data regarding their safety and efficacy in the pediatric population. Despite the almost explosive introduction of these agents into the marketplace over the past several decades, evaluation in the child has not proceeded concomitantly. Encouraging results from psychiatric drug usage in adults led to ready application of the same methods of therapy to children; stimulants, antidepressants, and tranquilizers are now being prescribed for children with various mental disorders. Although there has always been apprehension about using these drugs in children because of the possible permanent effects the drugs may have on later behavior, growth, and intelligence, there have been very few well-controlled studies which have established the safety, efficacy, dosage requirements, and disposition of this group of drugs in children.

Reasons for this gap in knowledge are manifold. Of utmost importance is the inability to diagnose and classify childhood mental illness. As a consequence, drug evaluation, even if attempted, has been carried out badly because of the nonrigorous nature of the clinical trial. Problems peculiar to drug evaluation in children, such as ethical considerations in minor subjects (especially if mentally retarded), have contributed to the lack of scientific data concerning psychotropic drug use in children. Other major factors responsible for the current status of pediatric psychopharmacology include the lack of pediatric clinical pharmacologists and the unavailability of adequate analytical methodology including micro methods, stable isotopes, and noninvasive approaches that would have facilitated drug evaluation in the minor subject.

Through repetitive use over the years, it has become evident that some drugs are of benefit to some children. Certain drugs (e.g., imipramine for enuresis, Poussaint et al., 1966; amphetamine for MBD, Conners, 1972) have been shown in placebo controlled studies definitely to be effective in illnesses peculiar to childhood. In general, however, determination of drug effectiveness has been very subjective.

Even more subjective have been the dosages prescribed to pediatric patients. Adjustment of the adult dose solely by body weight is inaccurate and has resulted in both toxicity and insufficient dosing of psychiatric drugs (Fish, 1968).

At the same time, impressive advances have occurred in our understanding of the action and disposition of psychotropics in adult patients: "steady-state" plasma and serum drug concentrations have been correlated in many instances with drug effects. Drug dosages have been modified to take into consideration patient variations in parameters such as rate of metabolism and elimination and extent of drug protein binding interaction with other drugs, as well as individual variation in drug response. The sophisticated and rational use of these compounds in the adult starkly contrasts with the empiric approach employed in the management of the sick infant and child.

The distribution and elimination of the psychoactive drugs in children may play a very important role in explaining differences seen in efficacy and safety between pediatric and adult patients. This is of particular significance with the psychoactive drugs because most of the drugs are highly bound to various body tissues (brain, liver, fat) and plasma proteins and have active metabolites (Byck, 1975). Although disposition of psychiatric drugs in children has not been studied, there have been many recent reports that drug disposition does differ with age. Antipyrine, phenylbutazone (Alvares et al., 1975), acetaminophen (Danish and Yaffe, 1975) and theophylline (Ellis, Levy, and Koysooko) are eliminated more rapidly in children. Protein binding may also change with age, since DPH protein binding has been shown to change during adolescence (Andritz and Jusko). In addition, children in general have less adipose tissue than adults.

Since assay methods are available for many of the psychoactive drugs, it is now possible to answer many of these questions concerning disposition in children. The ideal method for determining the correct dosage for children would come from measurement of drug concentrations at the presumed site of activity (e.g., CNS) and in the serum. This would be of great value in establishing a dose-serum-level-response curve.

Since this is not presently available it is necessary to use general pediatric guidelines for dosing and for measuring safety and efficacy.

Nonetheless, it is not too optimistic to consider that pediatric psychopharmacology will change with the acquisition of a data base from quality clinical trials. The classification which we have employed is predicated on this assumption.

Indeed, this book is an example of future trends in pediatric psychopharmacology with research formulations for the clinical use of these agents. Drugs have been characterized according to accepted use (psychoses, affective disorders, anxiety, and behavioral syndromes). Within each clinical situation further classification has been derived from chemical structure. Dosage recommendations in children have been purposefully not made since these are discussed in the individual chapters covering specific usage in children's mental illness. When disposition and pharmacodynamic data are available in children they are mentioned in addition to side effects and cautions which we think should be observed because of the stage of development of the child and the manner in which this may influence drug action and disposition.

ANTIPSYCHOTIC AGENTS

Three structural classes of psychotropic drugs are currently employed in the therapy of childhood and adolescent schizophrenia: The phenothiazines, the thioxanthenes, and the butyrophenones. Their pharmacologic properties, disposition, and side effects are discussed in the following paragraphs while their use in the psychotic child and adolescent is detailed in Chapter V.

1. The Phenothiazines

As a class, the phenothiazines are not only among the most widely used therapeutic agents but also appear to have the greatest array of pharmacologic effects, exerting an action on most organ systems. The phenothiazines consist of a triple-ring heterocyclic nucleus, in which two benzene rings are linked by both a sulfur and a nitrogen atom. Although many phenothiazine derivatives have been developed in the search for better antipsychotic medication, most are of equivalent potency.

The phenothiazines can be subdivided into three groups on the basis of substitution on the nitrogen atom in position ten in the middle ring. All substituted groups contain nitrogen, either in ring or chain form. Chlorpromazine, the most widely used and hence the prototype of the phenothiazines, has an aliphatic (aminoalkyl) side chain. Thiroidazine (Mellaril®), widely used as an adjunct in the management of the hyperactivity of psychotic children, is a member of the second group with a piperidine side chain. The other subgroup is the piperazine substituted group represented by prochlorperazine (Compazine®) and fluphen-azine (Prolixin®). All the phenothiazines used as antipsychotic agents have a three-carbon bridge between the nitrogen atom of the middle ring and that of the side chain. This is in contrast to the anticholinergic phenothiazines used in the management of parkinsonism and the antihistaminic phenothiazines that have only two carbons separating the nitrogen of the middle ring from the nitrogen of the side chain or ring.

The phenothiazines have diverse effects upon the central nervous system vary-ing from slowing of EEG patterns and increase in occurrence of theta waves to blockade of the chemoreceptor trigger zone of the medulla from the emetic ef-fects of apomorphine, a dopamine receptor stimulant. Considerable research has generated many hypotheses concerning the precise mechanism of action of the phenothiazines. The most attractive of these theories and the one which corre-lates well with antipsychotic activity involves blockade of dopamine mediated synaptic transmission (Matthysse, 1973). This mechanism may also explain how these drugs evoke parkinsonian-like extrapyramidal neurologic symptoms. Ani-mal studies have demonstrated that phenothiazines inhibit dopamine activation of adenylate cyclase in both the caudate nucleus and the limbic system. While this may be the dopamine receptor for the drug, the precise role of dopamine in the etiology of schizophrenia has not been established.

The disposition of the phenothiazines within the organism will depend upon the particular drug molecule. Chlorpromazine is discussed because of its wide-spread usage and thorough investigation. Peak plasma concentrations are found within several hours after oral administration. Elimination is almost entirely via hepatic metabolism into a large number of different metabolites. The plasma half-life of the parent drug is less than six hours but metabolites are excreted for weeks after cessation of administration. This is perhaps due to storage and dis-tribution in lipid, especially in the brain, where much higher concentrations are achieved than in plasma. There has been considerable research attempting to cor-relate blood concentrations with therapeutic response (Forrest, Carr, and Usdin, 1974). The 7-hydroxy derivative may correlate best with clinical effect. These correlations are confounded not only by the large numbers of metabolites but also by the fact that psychotic patients continue to show beneficial effects long after the drugs have been discontinued. More recently a specific sensitive GLC assay method for chlorpromazine has been developed (Rivera-Calimlin, Castaneda,

Lasagna, 1973). Improvement as determined by a psychiatric rating scale was found only in those patients with high plasma concentrations of 150–300 mg./ml. Patients with lower concentrations had no clinical improvement, while toxicity in the form of tremors and convulsions occurred with very high levels (750–1000 mg./ml.). While there are a few well-controlled studies of chlorpromazine efficacy in schizophrenic children at dosages of 2–9 mg./kg./day (Kurein et al., 1971), there are no studies of its disposition in the pediatric patient.

Since the many phenothiazine derivatives have similar clinical effects, the major differences relate to the nature and extent of side effects. Potency appears to increase from the piperidine to the aminoalkyl to the piperazine substituted drugs. Thus a continuum of side effects can be constructed with thioridazine at one end extending to chlorpromazine to perphenazine (Trilafon®) to fluphenazine. Sedation is greatest at the thioridazine end and least with fluphenazine, while neurologic effects are the opposite. These variations can be taken into consideration when patients manifest adverse effects. Granular deposits in the cornea have been seen in adult patients on very high doses of chlorpromazine. The major side effect of chronic administration is tardive dyskinesia (Marsden, Tarsy, and Baldessarani, 1975). These neurologic signs include athetoid movements of the hands, vermicular movements of the tongue, or tics of the lips or jaw. They are most often seen in older patients where drug metabolism may be altered. Cessation of therapy does not necessarily eliminate the adverse effects and the therapy may have to be continued, accepting the neurologic effects.

2. *The* Thioxanthenes

Thioxanthenes are structural derivatives of the phenothiazines with replacement of the nitrogen atom in the molecule at position ten by a carbon atom. Those thioxanthenes with central nervous system activity are characterized by a double bond between the C10 and the side chain as well as by substitutions in position two. While many thioxanthenes have been synthesized, only two are available for clinical use in the U.S.: chlorprothixene (Taractan®), an analogue of chlorpromazine, and thiothixene (Navane), an analogue of thioproperazine. It should be noted that because of a double bond at C10, two isomers of each substituted thioxanthene can be formed. These have been separated and the cis form is much more pharmacologically active than the trans isomer. Both thioxanthenes have actions similar to their phenothiazine analogues. While clinical studies of their efficacy abound, particularly in schizophrenic patients, there are no disposition data available. The studies of thiothixene in schizophrenic children are noteworthy because of the presence of antipsychotic activity without sedation, a major drawback with chlorpromazine therapy (Fish et al., 1969). A dosage of 6–30 mg./day (mean 14 mg./day) was efficacious in the management of ten psychotic boys aged five to fifteen years (Simeon et al., 1973). The improvement in behavior (emotional unresponsiveness, mood lability, attention span, motor activity, and socialization) correlated with improvement in EEG patterns. Extrapyramidal signs, one of the major adverse effects in adults, are less common in children.

3. Butyrophenones

While many *butyrophenones* have been synthesized and evaluated since the discovery of the neuroleptic and antipsychotic actions of this class, only two compounds are currently approved for use in the U.S.: haloperidol (Haldol®) and droperidol. The latter has a very short duration of action and is used only as an adjunct to general anesthesia. Although structurally different from the phenothiazines, the butyrophenones share many of their pharmacologic properties. Haloperidol is an extremely potent antipsychotic shown to be effective both in the treatment of manic illness and in schizophrenia. Its mechanism of action is considered to be similar to the phenothiazines since it also blocks the effects of dopamine.

Haloperidol has been extensively used in child psychiatry. Two studies have compared its effectiveness with that of fluphenazine in schizophrenic children. In one investigation haloperidol in doses up to 16 mg./day was successful in reducing autism and provocative behavior (Faretra, Dooher, and Dowling, 1970). In the other study there were considerably fewer extrapyramidal side effects with haloperidol than with the phenothiazines (Engelhardt et al., 1973).

The disposition of the drug is unknown in children. Studies in man are incomplete. The drug appears to be rapidly absorbed from the gastrointestinal tract with peak plasma concentrations reached at two hours. Elimination occurs only after metabolism in the liver. It is important to note that no correlation was found between therapeutic response and plasma concentration of the parent drug (Zingales, 1971).

Side effects appear to be dose related and on the whole consist of extrapyramidal reactions. These were of a low incidence in the two pediatric studies cited above.

STIMULANTS

The pediatric clinical syndromes of hyperkinesis or minimal brain dysfunction are characterized by motor restlessness, impulsiveness, learning difficulty and a low frustration tolerance (Eisenberg, 1972). Although not all children benefit from stimulant drug therapy, and the use of stimulants in children is controversial, controlled studies have shown the efficacy of stimulants in certain children and a four- to eight-week trial period of drug therapy is often worthwhile. The stimulants most often employed are dextramphetamine, methylphenidate, and pemoline. A more complete discussion of their use in minimal brain dysfunction is included in ch. six.

1. Amphetamine

Amphetamines have been used for almost forty years in the treatment of children with behavior disorders (Bradley, 1937). Amphetamines are sympathomimetic phenylethylamines that are powerful CNS stimulants, in addition to having peripheral alpha and beta adrenergic activity. The d-isomer has greater CNS effects and fewer cardiovascular effects than the 1-isomer and is the form most often administered to children.

The mechanism of action of amphetamines in behavioral disorders has not been clearly identified. Amphetamines do act to promote the release and prevent the reuptake of monamines from the neurons; it is probably through this effect on CNS neurotransmitters that amphetamines enhance the functioning of the reticular activating system and thereby improve the behavior reinforcement system mediated through cortical inhibition (Snyder, 1973; Baldessarani, 1972).

Amphetamines are readily absorbed after oral administration and are rapidly distributed to tissues, especially kidney, lung, and brain (Maikel et al., 1969). The half-life of amphetamine has been reported to be approximately five hours in adults with an acidic urine (Beckett, 1969). Serum half-life increases with chronic use. About 35 to 40 percent of amphetamine is excreted unchanged in an alkaline pH; an acidic urine increases excretion of the unchanged drug to 70 percent (Anggard, 1970). Amphetamine is metabolized by two major pathways in man, oxidative deamination and hydroxylation. It has been suggested that the hydroxylation pathway is responsible for production of false neurotransmitters and that these metabolites are retained in the body longer than the parent drug.

There have been no studies done in hyperkinetic children to determine if there are differences from adults in the disposition of the drug. However, Epstein et al., (1968) have monitored urinary excretion of dextroamphetamine and found a higher percentage of unchanged drug in the responders as compared to nonresponders at seven hours after administration. Further studies are needed to determine if hyperkinesis or the age of the patient affects drug metabolism.

Side effects are reported in approximately 10 to 15 percent of children taking amphetamines, but they are usually not serious enough to warrant discontinuation (Millichap and Fowler, 1967). The most serious effect is psychosis with hallucinations. The degree of psychosis has been directly related to the concentration of the hydroxylated amphetamine metabolites in the urine (Anggard et al., 1973). Although rare, psychosis has been reported in children (Ney, 1967).

Anorexia and weight loss are common at doses greater than 15 mg./day (Fish, 1968), but tolerance to these effects and to the insomnia usually develops within one to two weeks. Chronic administration may suppress growth and this should be carefully monitored.

Dizziness, irritability, cardiac arrhythmias, and nausea and vomiting have been observed after accidental ingestion.

Long-term safety in children has not been ascertained. This is of particular importance with drugs that effect the CNS and are used for months to years during a period of continuous brain development and maturation.

2. Methylphenidate

Methylphenidate is a piperidine derivative of amphetamine. The pharmacological and behavioral properties are essentially the same as amphetamine (Martin et al., 1971). Methylphenidate is at least equally effective (Conners, 1971) and possibly more effective (Millichap and Fowler, 1967) than dextroamphetamine in the treatment of hyperkinetic children.

The metabolic fate of methylphenidate in man has not yet been elucidated. However, methylphenidate may influence the metabolism of other drugs, including the anticonvulsants (Garretson, 1969).

Side effects are seen in about 14 percent of children treated with methylphenidate (Millichap and Fowler, 1967). This is similar to the percentage of side effects seen with dextroamphetamine; however, there is probably less suppression of weight gain with methylphenidate (Safer et al., 1972). Acute episodes of psychosis and hallucinations have also been reported with methylphenidate (Lucas and Weiss, 1971).

3. Pemoline

Magnesium pemoline is an oxazolidine derivative which has been introduced into pediatrics as an alternative to the amphetamine-like drugs for treatment of hyperkinesis. Its chemical structure differs from amphetamine and methyphenidate and it has no sympathomimetic activity.

Pemoline is a CNS stimulant and although its mechanism of action in man is not known, it does increase dopamine synthesis in the rat brain (Tagliamonte et al., 1971).

The half-life of pemoline averages twelve hours and once-a-day dosing is usually sufficient. In two placebo controlled studies (Conners, 1972; Page et al., 1974), pemoline was reported effective in treating MBD, with the maximum response observed after six weeks of therapy.

The reported side effects have been most often related to the drug's CNS stimulatory effects: anorexia, insomnia, restlessness, dizziness, and headaches (Page et al., 1974). Initial weight loss has been reported to return to the normal weight-gain curve after three to six months of drug administration. Psychosis has been reported in adults after chronic administration. There have been no long-term studies of pemoline's effect on growth and until such data become available, the growth rate should be monitored in all patients.

ANTIDEPRESSANTS

1. The Tricyclic Antidepressants

The tricyclic antidepressants, represented by imipramine (Tofranil®), amitryptyline (Elavil®), and their demethylated metabolites, desipramine and nortriptyline, are used in the treatment of children with depression, hyperactive-aggressive behavior and enuresis.

The mechanism of action of these drugs in the management of any of these conditions has not been ascertained. However, it is known that the tricyclics inhibit the neuronal uptake of monoamines. It has been theorized that depression may be caused by insufficient quantities of norepinephrine or serotonin at CNS receptor sites and by preventing the reuptake of norepinephrine and serotonin by the nerve terminal, more of these amines are available at the presumed site of activity. Although it is known that the demethylated tricyclics are more potent in the blockade of norepinephrine and the methylated drugs are more effective in the blockade of serotonin reuptake, the clinical significance of this differential is not clear. It has also been demonstrated that in animals higher doses of tricyclics may actually antagonize the effects of norepinephrine on the adrenergic receptors (Haefely et al., 1964) which may partially account for the side effects seen with the tricyclics at higher doses (Sjoqvist et al., 1971).

The mechanism by which the tricyclics act in enuresis is even less well understood. It has been postulated that in addition to their effect on mood, their anticholinergic and central stimulant properties may play a role in alleviating enuresis (Poussaint et al., 1966).

The tricyclics are rapidly and completely absorbed after oral administration. However, only 29 to 77 percent of imipramine (Gram and Christiansen, 1975) and 46 to 60 percent of nortriptyline (Gram and Overo, 1975) are systemically available because the drugs are metabolized in the liver before entering the general systemic circulation (first pass effect).

It requires two to three weeks of daily therapy to see a therapeutic response to the tricyclics. This corresponds to the duration of time needed to reach steady state plasma levels because of long half-lives. (Imipramine half-lives in children vary from twenty-five to sixty hours) (Winsberg et al., 1974).

Steady state plasma levels show large variations in patients on equivalent doses (Sjoqvist et al., 1971). This can be attributed to variance in the rate of metabolism and, to a lesser extent, differences in protein binding. The rate of metabolism is genetically determined and may also be effected by exposure to other drugs (Alexanderson et al., 1969).

It is the amount of free drug which is considered the active component available at the site of action. Therefore, the protein binding of imipramine, which changes with age, may be very important in determining dosage requirements: 26 percent is free in the neonate, 14 to 22 percent in the seven- to ten-year-old group and 5 to 23 percent free in depressed adult patients (Winsberg et al., 1974).

The tricyclics are fat soluble and have a large volume of distribution (about 15 to 30 liters/kg. in the adult) (Sjoqvist et al., 1971). Children generally have smaller adipose compartments than adults, and this may increase the amount of drug available to the CNS (Winsberg et al., 1974).

In adults, the tricyclics have an overall adverse reaction rate of 15 percent while major adverse reactions (psychosis, hallucinations, etc.) occur in 4.6 percent (Boston Collaborative Drug Surveillance Program, 1972). The most commonly reported complaints are related to the anticholinergic effects of the drugs and include dry mouth, decreased gut motility, and urinary retention.

In addition to the anticholinergic effects, the tricyclics do have an affinity for cardiac tissue and may cause a direct myocardial depression. Other cardiovascular findings include a decreased cardiac output and an increased duration of the QRS complex on electrocardiograms (Thorstrand, 1974).

In summary, the tricyclic antidepressants are useful drugs in children, especially for the treatment of enuresis. The disposition studies done in children illustrate the importance of determining dose-response relationships in this age group and the error that can occur from extrapolation from adult data. Since the safety and efficacy of various suggested dosage regimens for children have not been thoroughly studied, children should be carefully monitored while receiving medication, particularly with long-term administration. Doses of 1–2 mg./kg./day have been established for enuresis. While higher doses have been used as an antidepressant, doses above this may be unsafe and should be carefully monitored for electrocardiographic abnormalities.

2. The MAO Inhibitors

The monoamine oxidase (MAO) inhibitors include the hydrazide derivatives: isocarboxacid, nialamide, and phenelzine; and the nonhydrazides, tranylcypromine and pargyline, have been used in the past for the treatment of depression and narcolepsy. Because of the high potential for toxicity and the disputed efficacy of this group of drugs, their use in recent years has greatly diminished. However, the MAO inhibitors do offer an alternative method of therapy for patients with atypical endogenous depression which does not respond to the drugs of choice, the tricyclics (Johnson, 1975).

The monomine oxidase enzymes are located primarily within the neuron and are major regulators of epinephrine, norepinephrine, dopamine, and serotonin metabolism. The MAO inhibitors irreversibly inactivate the isoenzymes that deaminate the monoamines and allow an increase in intracellular amine levels. The correlation of their psychological effects with this physiological effect has not yet been demonstrated despite considerable research effort. The MAO inhibitors, particularly phenelzine and tranylcypromine, have been reported to elevate the mood of depressed patients and suppress REM sleep. As with the tricyclics, it takes several weeks of daily administration for a response to be observed; this is probably because their activity depends upon the rate of enzyme synthesis. Prospective studies still are needed to evaluate their role in pediatric psychiatry.

The MAO inhibitors are lipophilic compounds which are absorbed from the gut and readily cross the blood-brain barrier. The hydrazide derivatives are thought to be cleaved before activation. Phenelzine is probably dehydrazinated to phenylacetic acid by an MAO catalyzed reaction (Horita et al., 1969). The nonhydrazine group combines directly with the MAO isoenzymes and unlike the hydrazide group, this union may be slowly reversible. The hydrazide group is deactivated by acetylation; about half the adult population are slow acetylators of phenelzine, which may effect the observed response to the drug (Johnstone and Marsh 1973).

The toxicity reported with the MAO inhibitors has been the major factor responsible for decreased use of these drugs. Although all the drugs in this group can potentially cause severe adverse reactions, the two drugs now in common use, phenelzine and tranylcypromine, rarely cause any serious problems at therapeutic dosage levels (Raskin, 1972).

With an acute overdose, symptoms occur in a few hours and can usually be characterized by agitation, hallucinations, hyperpyrexia, convulsions, and occasionally coma and death. Both increases and decreases in blood pressure are observed. Dialysis may be of value in decreasing the serum levels (Matter et al., 1965).

Hepatotoxicity, which is not dose related, has been reported in patients on chronic therapy. Other side effects reported with long-term therapy include tremors, insomnia, peripheral neuropathy, and orthostatic hypotension (Byck, 1975). Less serious complaints have included headaches, dizziness, fatigue, constipation, and urinary retention.

The various cardiovascular and autonomic side effects observed with MAO inhibitor administration are usually tolerable; however, a greater possibility for toxicity occurs in their interaction with food and other drugs. MAO inhibitors potentiate the effect of peripherally acting amines, particularly amphetamines and tyramine. It is of utmost importance to alert patients to this interaction because a hypertensive crisis may occur if the patient ingests food products containing tyramine (cheeses, beer, wines, liver, pickled herring, tripe, yeast, coffee, canned figs or large portions of any dairy product) (Marley and Blackwell, 1970).

MAO inhibitors also inhibit liver enzymes other than MAO and therefore could inhibit the metabolism of anesthetics, barbiturates, and narcotics (Eade and Renton, 1970).

In summary, the administration of MAO inhibitors to children should be approached with extreme caution because of the lack of data in children and the reported adverse reactions in adults.

TRANQUILIZERS

A number of different classes of pharmacologic agents are used in children with anxiety and neurotic symptoms. The drugs most frequently prescribed are the benzodiazepines (diazepam, chlordiazepoxide, clorazepate, flurazepam and oxazepam) and the antihistamine sedatives (hydroxyzine and diphenhydramine). The propanediol carbamates, meprobamate, and tybamate are used so rarely (and for other indications) as not to warrant discussion.

The benzodiazepines have been the subject of a recent review (Greenblatt and Shader, 1974). They are extremely widely used, but no data are available concerning age distribution of usage. Thirty percent of medical inpatients in the Boston teaching hospitals monitored by the Boston Collaborative Drug Surveillance Program in 1973 received diazepam and 32 percent flurazepam. Outpatient usage is just as frequent; 77 million prescriptions were filled in retail pharmacies in 1972.

The various benzodiazepine derivatives have qualitatively similar properties despite variations in potency. The behavioral effects seen in animals following benzodiazepine administration have been collectively termed ''disinhibition.'' These include an increase in spontaneous and exploratory activity, suppression of behavior motivated by punishment, and attenuation of the behavioral sequelae of stress. These are mentioned because clinical antianxiety effects of drugs are speculated to be the counterpart of ''disinhibition'' in animals. These procedures are used for screening and development of new compounds. It is noteworthy that behavioral effects in animals produced by the benzodiazepines occur at low dosages, whereas nonspecific central nervous system depression requires much larger dosages. Although meprobamate and barbiturates also produce ''disinhibition," they do so at doses very close to toxicity. The major tranquilizers (see under antipsychotic agents) do not produce "disinhibition" in animals at any dose.

Diazepam is rapidly absorbed following oral administration with a peak level occurring at two hours. The intramuscular route should not be used because of very erratic absorption. The drug is slowly metabolized to the desmethyl derivative (half-life of one to two days). This active compound is subsequently hydroxylated (oxazepam) and rapidly glucuronidated before renal excretion. Steady state concentrations are reached about a week after initiation of therapy. Diazepam disposition in children is somewhat more rapid than in adults with a plasma half-life of eighteen hours (Morselli et al., 1973). Because of the relatively slow rates of metabolism, diazepam and chlordiazepoxide can be given one to two times a day. Oxazepam with a rapid biotransformation to inactive metabolites requires three to four doses per day. The slowly metabolized compounds tend to accumulate, with clinical effects or toxicity not apparent until seven to ten days after the initiation of therapy. Similarly, effects may be evident for some time after the cessation of therapy. These pharmacokinetic properties must be kept in mind when dosages are altered. Toxic reactions and side effects are minimal with these compounds. This undoubtedly has played a major role in their widespread usage. Drowsiness, the most common side effect, is an extension of the pharmacologic action and can be eliminated by reduction of dosage.

The antihistamine sedatives continue to be used in pediatric practice. Diphenhydramine (Benadry®) is effective in young children as an antianxiety agent irrespective of the presence of hyperactivity (Fish and Shapiro, 1965). At puberty effectiveness decreases and an increase in dose is associated with drowsiness. For this reason, it is used as a bedtime sedative in this age group. The efficacy of hydroxyzine (Atarax®) in the management of anxiety is less clear. There are conflicting reports as to whether or not it is better than a placebo in adult subjects. There are, however, no studies reported in children and usage in this age group cannot be recommended (*Medical Letter*, 1970).

SUMMARY *

The use of psychoactive agents in adults has been followed by their application in children, without consideration or resolution of the special problems of drug administration to this age group. These problems include the difficulty of accurate

* Editor's summary.

or agreed-upon diagnosis, the effects on later growth and development, ethical considerations, and inadequate analytical methodology. Compared to studies in adults, little is known about site mechanism of action, the pharmacokinetics, efficacy variations, or dosage rationale for these drugs in children. There is reason to believe that drug disposition in children is different from that in adults, and the results of drug-serum-level-response studies should be forthcoming as a basis for determining efficacy and dosage.

Drugs are classified according to accepted clinical use and within each clinical situation by chemical structure.

The antipsychotic agents include the phenothiazines, thioxanthenes, and butyrophenones. The phenothiazines, differing in side effects by aliphatic, piperidine, and piperezine side chains, most likely act by blockade of dopamine mediated synaptic transmission. There are no studies of phenothiazine disposition in children, although their efficacy in schizophrenic children has been demonstrated at doses of 2–9 mg./kg./day.

The thioxanthenes are chemically related to the phenothiazines, but provide antipsychotic activity without as much sedation.

The butyrophenones, primarily haloperidol, are structurally different from the phenothiazines, but have potent antipsychotic properties, also apparently acting by dopamine blockade, but with fewer extrapyramidal side effects.

The stimulant drugs include the amphetamines, methylphenidate, and pemoline. The amphetamines and methylphenidate promote release and prevent reuptake of monoamines, probably in this way enhancing the functioning of the reticular activating system. Ready absorption after oral intake, rapid distribution to kidney, lung, and brain, and urinary excretion characterize their disposition. Anorexia, weight loss, and insomnia are the more common side effects; psychosis with hallucinations is a rare occurrence.

The tricyclic antidepressants inhibit the neuronal uptake of monoamines, making these neurotransmitters more available at receptor sites. They are metabolized by the liver with wide variations in plasma levels on equivalent doses. Free levels in the plasma decrease with age, and this may be related to dosage decisions. So far, the major use of the tricyclics in children has been the administration of imipramine for enuresis. Its mechanism of action in this symptom, possibly related to its anticholinergic properties, has not been actually defined. Its use as an antidepressant in children is still unclear. In higher doses potentially dangerous cardiovascular effects may occur and indicate cautious usage.

Although much is known about the mechanism of action and disposition of the MAO inhibitors in adults, their high potential for toxicity, absence of documented advantage to the tricyclics, and lack of data in children should severely limit their use in this age group.

The benzodiazepines are increasingly more widely used, but there are no data regarding usage by age distribution, mechanism of action, efficacy, or indications for use in children. They are characterized by rapid absorption, a half-life of eighteen hours in children, low toxicity, and few side effects, all of which make them attractive agents.

It should be reemphasized that the conditions for an adequate pharmacology and classification of psychoactive agents in childhood have yet to be met, namely data regarding mechanism and site of action, pharmacodynamics, and disposition. Until then, classification remains largely clinical, dosage primarily experiential, and results determined empirically.

References

Alexanderson, B., Sjoqvist, F., and Price-Evans, D. (1969), Steady state plasma levels of nor-triptyline in twins: influence of genetic factors and drug therapy. *Brit. Med. J., 4,* 764.

Alvares, A. P., Kapeliner, S., Sassa, S., and Kappas, A. (1975), Drug metabolism in normal children, lead poisoned children, and normal adults. *Clin. Pharm. Ther., 17,* 179.

Andritz, M. and Jusko, W., Personal communication.

Anggard, E., Gunner, L., Jonsson, L., and Niklasson, F. (1970), Pharmacokinetic and clinical studies on amphetamine dependent subjects. *Eur. J. Clin. Pharm., 3,* 3.

Anggard, E., Jonsson, L., Hogmark, A., and Gunne, L. (1973), Amphetamine metabolism in amphetamine psychosis. *Clin. Pharm. Ther., 14,* 870.

Baldessarani, R. J. (1972), Pharmacology of the amphetamines. *Pediatrics,* pp. 49–694.

Beckett, A. H. (1969), Drug metabolism and kinetics of sympathomimetic amines in man. In A. Cerletti, and F. Bove (Eds.), *The present status of psychotropic drugs*. Excerpta Med. Found.

Boston Collaborative Drug Surveillance Program (1972), Adverse reactions to the tricyclic antidepressant drugs. *Lancet, 1,* 529.

Bradley, C. (1937), The behavior of children receiving Benzedrine. *Amer. J. Psychiat., 94,* 577.

Byck, R. (1975), Drugs and the treatment of psychiatric disorders. In L. S. Goodman, and A. Gilman (Eds.), *The pharmacological basis of therapeutics*, Fifth Ed. New York; Macmillan.

Conners, C. K. (1971), Recent drug studies with hyperkinetic children. *J. Learn. Disabil., 4,* 476.

Conners, C. K. (1972), Psychological effects of stimulant drugs in children with minimal brain dysfunction. *Pediatrics, 49,* 702.

Danish, M. and Yaffe, S. (1975), Acetaminophen disposition in adolescents. *Ped. Res.* (abst.), *9,* 283.

Eade, N. R., and Renton, K. W. (1970), The effect of phenelzine and tranylcypromine on the degradation of meperidine. *J. Pharm. Exp. Ther., 173,* 31–36.

Eisenberg, L. (1972), The clinical use of stimulant drugs in children. *Pediatrics, 49,* 709.

Ellis, E. F., Levy, G., and Koysooko, R. Pharmacokinetics of theophylline in children. Submitted for publication.

Engelhardt, D. M., Polizoes, P., Waizer, J., and Hoffman, S. P. (1973), A double-blind comparison of fluphenazine and haloperidol in out-patient schizophrenic children. *J. Aut. & Ch. Schiz., 3,* 127–128.

Epstein, L. C., Lasagna, L., and Conners, C. K. (1968), Correlation of dextroamphetamine excretion and drug response in hyperkinetic children. *J. Nerv. Ment. Dis., 146,* 136.

Faretra, G., Dooher, C., and Dowling, J. (1970), Comparison of haloperidol and fluphenazine in disturbed children. *Am. J. Psychiat., 126,* 146–149.

Fish, B. (1968), Drug therapy in children's psychiatric disorders. In F. A. Freyhan, N. Petrelowitsch, and P. Pichot, (Eds.), *Modern problems of pharmacopsychiatry*. Basel: Vol. 1, p. 60.

Fish, B., and Shapiro, T. (1965), A typology of children's psychiatric disorders: Its application to a controlled evaluation of treatment. *J. Amer. Acad. Ch. Psychiat., 4,* 32–52.

Fish, B., Campbell, M., Shapiro, T., and Weinstein, J. (1969), Preliminary findings on thiothixene compared to other drugs in psychotic children. In H. E. Lehmaix, and T. A. Ban Karger (Eds.), *The thioxanthenes: Modern problems of pharmacopsychiatry*. Basel 2, 90–99.

Forrest, I. S., Carr, C. J., and Usdin, E. (1974), *Phenothiazines and structurally related drugs*. New York: Raven Press.

Garretson, L. K., Perel, J. M., and Dayton, P. G. (1969), Methylphenidate interaction with both anticonvulsants and ethylbiscoumacetate. *J.A.M.A., 207,* 2052.

Gram, L., and Christiansen, J. (1975), First pass metabolism of imipramine in man. *Clin. Pharm. Ther., 17,* 555.

Gram, L., and Overo, K. (1975), First pass metabolism of nortriptyline in man. *Clin. Pharm. Ther., 18,* 305.

Greenblatt, D. J., and Shader, R. I. (1974), Benzodiazepines. *N.E.J.M., 291,* 1011–1015.

Haefely, W., Hurlimann, A., and Thoesen, H. (1964), Scheenbar paradoxe beeinflussung von peripheren noradrenaliniverkungen durch einige thymoleptika. *Helv. Physiol. Acta, 22,* 15.

Horita, A., Clineschmidt, B. V., and McMonigle, J. J. (1969), The role of metabolism in the action of some monoamine oxidase inhibitors. In A. Cerletti, and F. J. Bove (Eds.), *The present status of psychotropic drugs*. Excerpta Med. Found.

Johnson, W. C. (1975), A neglected modality in psychiatric treatment—the monoamine oxidase inhibitors. *Dis. Nerv. Sys.,* p. 521.

Johnstone, E. C., and Marsh, W. (1973), Acetylator status and response to phenelzine in depressed patients. *Lancet, 1,* 567.

Kurein, J., Fish, B., Shapiro, T., Gerner, E. W., and Levidow, C. (1971), EEG and behavioral effects of drug therapy in children: Chlorpromazine and diphenhydramine. *Arch. Gen. Psychiat., 24,* 552.

Lucas, A. R., and Weiss, M. (1971), Methylphenidate hallucinosis. *J.A.M.A., 217,* 1079.

Maikel, R. P., Cox, R. H., Miller, F. P., Segal, D. S., and Russell, R. W. (1969), Correlation of brain levels of drugs with behavioral effects. *J. Pharm. Exp. Ther., 165,* 216.

Marley, E., and Blackwell, B. (1970), Interactions of monoamine oxidase inhibitors, amines and foodstuffs. *Adv. Pharma. Chemother., 8,* 185.

Marsden, D. C., Tarsy, D., and Baldessarani, R. J. (1975), Spontaneous and drug induced movement disorders in psychotic patients. In D. F. Benson, and D. Blumer (Eds.), *Psychiatric complications of neurological diseases*. New York: Grune and Stratton.

Martin, W. R., Sloan, J. W., Sapira, J. D., and Jasinski, D. R. (1971), Physiologic, subjective and behavioral effects of amphetamine, methamphetamine, ephedrine, phenmetrazine and methylphenidate in man. *Clin. Pharm. Ther.,* pp. 12–245.

Matter, B. J., Donat, P. E., Brill, M. L., and Ginn, H. F. (1965), Tranylcypromine sulfate poisoning. *Arch. Int. Med.,* pp. 116–18.

Matthysse, S. (1973), Antipsychotic drug actions: A clue to the neuropathology of schizophrenia. *Fed. Proc., 32,* 200.

Medical Letter (1970), *18,* 74.

Millichap, J. G., and Fowler, G. W. (1967), Treatment of "minimal brain dysfunction" syndromes. *Ped. Clin. N. Amer., 14,* 767.

Morselli, P. L., Principi, N., Tognoni, G., Reali, E., Belvedere, G., Standen, S. M., and Sereni, F. (1973), Diazepam elimination in premature and full term infants and children. *J. Perinat. Med., 1,* 133.

Ney, P. G. (1967), Psychosis in a child, associated with amphetamine administration. *Canad. Med. Assn. J., 97,* 1026.

Page, J. G., Bernstein, J. E., Janicki, R. S., and Michelli, F. A. (1974), A multi-clinic trial of permoline in childhood hyperkinesis. In C. K. Conners (Ed.), *The clinical use of stimulant drugs in children*. Excerpta Med.

Poussaint, A. F., Ditman, K., and Greenfield, R. (1966), Amtriptyline in childhood enuresis. *Clin. Pharm. Ther., 7,* 21.

Raskin, A. (1972), Adverse reactions to phenelzine: Results of a nine-hospital depression study. *J. Clin. Pharmacol., 12,* 22.

Rivera-Calimlin, L., Castaneda, L., and Lasagna, L. (1973), Effects of mode of management on plasma chlorpromazine in psychiatric patients. *Clin. Pharmacol. Ther., 14,* 978.

Safer, D., Allen R., and Barr, E. (1972), Depression of growth in hyperactive children on stimulant drugs. *N.E.J.M., 287,* 217.

Simeon, J., Saletu, B., Saletu, M., Itil, T. M., and DaSilva, J. (1973), Thiothixine in childhood psychoses. Presented at third international Symposium on Phenothiazines, Rockville, Maryland.

Sjoqvist, F., Alexanderson, B., Asberg, M., Bertilsson, L., Borga, O., Hamberger, B. and Tuck, D. (1971), Pharmacokinetics and biological effects of nortriptyline in man. *Acta Pharm. Toxicol., 29* (Suppl. 3), 255.

Synder, S. H. (1973), How amphetamine acts in minimal brain dysfunction. *Acad. Sci., 205,* 310.

Tagliamonte, A. P., Tagliamonte, J., Perez-Cruet, and Geasa, G. L. (1971), Stimulation of brain dopamine turnover by magnesium pemoline. *Fed. Proc., 30,* 223, (abst.).

Thorstrand, C. (1974), Cardiovascular effects of poisoning with tricyclic antidepressants. *Acta Med. Scand., 195,* 205.

Winsberg, B. G., Perel, J., Hurivic, M., and Klutch, A. (1974), Imipramine protein binding and pharmacokinetics in children. In I. S. Forrest, C. J. Carr, and E. Usdin (Eds.), *The phenothiazines and structurally related drugs.* New York: Raven Press.

Zingales, I. A. (1971), A gas chromatographic method for the determination of haloperidol in human plasma. *J. Chromatography, 54,* 15.

Chapter Three

METHODOLOGICAL CONSIDERATIONS IN DRUG RESEARCH WITH CHILDREN

C. Keith Conners, PH.D.

Drug research with children has shown a steady increase in quantity over the past ten years (Lipman, 1974), and with this increase has come a greater sophistication and critical approach to methodological problems. Many of these problems are identical to those found in psychopharmacology with adults, but much of the content of documentation is specific to children and special problems encountered in such research include: diagnosis and selection of subjects for a drug trial; measurement of dependent variables; research design; ethical considerations; nondrug variables such as developmental level and changes over time associated with changing development status of the child; and interactions with other treatments.

Many of these issues have been addressed by the American Academy of Pediatrics (1975), and a recent task force of the FDA has developed more specific guidelines and recommendations covering Phase I, II, and III drug trials with children. A special issue of the *Psychopharmacology Bulletin* dealing with drug studies in children (NIMH 1973) contains many important contributions to the area including measuring instruments which have been adopted by the Early Clinical Drug Evaluation Unit (ECDEU) of the National Institute of Mental Health. A publication entitled "Documentation of Clinical Psychotropic Drug Trials" published by the Psychopharmacology Branch of NIMH sets out a complete documentation system for drug trials which should prove valuable to any investigator desiring a comprehensive and systematic format for drug investigations with children.

DIAGNOSIS AND SELECTION OF SUBJECTS

It is a truism that diagnositc categories in childhood psychiatric disturbances are less precise, theoretically more uncertain and empirically less validated than in adult disorders. Careful consideration of diagnostic issues has been given in several excellent sources and should be consulted prior to drug trials with children (Group for Advancement of Psychiatry, 1966; Werry, 1973; Knights, 1973; Rutter et al., 1969; Klein and Gittelman-Klein, 1974; Fish and Shapiro, 1965). Regardless of the investigator's theoretical biases, there are a number of essential criteria which should be met in the diagnostic evaluation used in a particular drug study; these have been outlined by Werry (1973) as follows:

1. The system should be acceptable to most investigators—simple, topical, comprehensible, accurate, and useful.
2. It should specify the data domain and the method of eliciting the data. This domain should be wide enough to cover all conditions, including uncommon ones like psychosis.
3. The decision flow from data to diagnosis should be explicated.
4. Diagnoses should be mutually exclusive. This does not preclude making a secondary diagnosis. It just means that one set of data should lead to a clear terminal diagnostic point distinct from all others.
5. Diagnosis should be reliable across investigators.
6. Diagnosis should be valid in predicting drug responders and meaningful in terms of current concepts and theory and in describing samples of children studied.
7. Diagnoses should be in a form suitable for statistical analysis, i.e., capable of being reduced to numbers or scales rather than a purely descriptive statement.

In general, to meet these criteria one must specify the types of data used to arrive at the diagnosis (e.g., interview, history, symptoms reported or observed), and relate these data explicitly to the necessary and sufficient criteria established for the diagnosis. For example, the DSM II (1968) category for *Schizophrenia, Childhood Type* (295.8), subcategory Autism, provides a comprehensive list of symptoms, signs, and behaviors under "Necessary and Sufficient Symptoms," "Symptoms Commonly Associated But Not Sufficient for Diagnosis," and "Disqualifiers."

Data for this diagnosis could include (a) direct observation of the child; (b) verbal reports from the child; (c) data obtained from history or informants. In each case, the specific symptoms required should be spelled out and the procedure for establishing the reliability of the observations explicitly indicated. For the psychiatric interview this process can be greatly facilitated by use of a formal rating scale whose reliability has been established under standard conditions. One example of such a scale has been used by Rutter and colleagues (1968). This system clearly defines which symptoms are rated on direct observations as opposed to verbal report. If symptoms are included from parents, teachers, or other informants, the method of ascertaining these, as well as their reliability, should be indicated. If the *severity* of a symptom enters into the diagnosis (e.g., "gross impairment"), the cutoff scale point needs to be specified (e.g., severity rating greater than five on a nine-point scale). It is also important to note that disqualifiers as well as commonly associated but not sufficient symptoms are useful. In this way, regardless of another investigator's difference of opinion on theoretical issues, the procedures for selecting and defining the target population for the study can be replicated or placed in a different diagnostic framework if desired.

Reliability is a central issue in all measurement and can be arrived at in a number of different ways. A co-observer can observe the same interview, use a recorded version from the initial interview, reinterview the child at a different time, or use a different basis for the diagnosis altogether. Reliabilities from these approaches will often differ so that the particular method employed should be made explicit. Typically, symptoms such as anxiety, depression, and mood present difficulties in obtaining satisfactory reliabilities unless quite precise definitions are used. Recent work by Englehardt and Gittelman-Klein (unpublished) has shown that the Child Psychiatric Rating Scale from the ECDEU battery can produce quite satisfactory reliabilities, thus providing a powerful tool for complex integrative measures such as diagnosis.

The purposes of accurate diagnosis are to establish homogeneous samples and to facilitate comparisons and communication with the work of other investigators. Some will argue that diagnosis is a futile exercise and that reliable, valid target symptoms or dimensional continua are sufficient. My own opinion is that diagnostic formulations provide important heuristic, communication, and theoretical advantages within the broader context of psychiatric research, and that most dimensional systems can be reduced to diagnostic categories by specifying the translation rules, cutting points and data domains from which the symptoms or continua are drawn. Careful discussion of these issues will be found in Werry (1973).

MEASUREMENT OF DEPENDENT VARIABLES IN DRUG RESEARCH

The purpose for using psychoactive drugs in children, after all, is to alter favorably symptoms or behavior. The adequate assessment of efficacy requires methods for both reliable and valid documentation of change associated with drug administration. Along with precisely defined study populations, discussed above in this chapter and by Werry (1973), the measurement of change (dependent variable) is a sine qua non of drug research. Only in the past few years have there been available more objective and replicable measurement methods. Because of the recent developments in this field and the complexities in design of several of the instruments which have been developed, this section will go into relatively more detail by way of discussing the methods now available. Those methods include direct observation, behavior rating scales, performance and laboratory measures, neuro-developmental measures, projective type measures, and measurement of side effects and toxicity.

A. Direct Observational Methods

Direct methods of measuring a child's behavior have several advantages in drug research: the specific behaviors being monitored can usually be obtained repeatedly over time without interfering with the behavior; the target behavior can be precisely defined and reliably measured; the validity of the measure is usually unambiguous (e.g., "time on task" in a classroom carries a clear indication of the meaning of the datum); and discrete components of behavior can be analyzed in relation to less direct methods such as ratings, and compared with other behaviors of clinical interest to elucidate the degree and range of drug effect. A thorough treatment of direct methods can be found in recent publications (Mann, 1976; Doke, 1976).

The essential features of direct measurement systems are: (a) a precise definition of the behavior in directly observable form; (b) explicit rules for the time and place of recording; (c) establishing satisfactory observer reliability; (d) sufficient replication of observations to obtain a stable baseline; (e) observation and recording of the behavior with and without drug treatment to determine drug effects. An illustration of such an approach can be given with a system modified from Monkman (1972) as applied by this author in an impatient setting for children. Figure 1 shows data on a twelve-year-old boy admitted to the hospital because of severe antisocial behavior, including aggressive behavior with peers. The data are based upon sixteen minutes of interval time sampling of interactions each day, collected in four-minute periods at four different periods of the day. There appears to be a clear and unequivocal improvement in the percent of positive peer interactions during the course of hospitalization after the introduction of treatment with methylphenidate. The observers had been trained to a high degree of reliability (0.90 or better) and were unaware of the treatment condition. It should be noted that although such a finding is suggestive, the simple A-B design leaves open the possibility that the effect was due to a placebo phenomenon, to spontaneous improvement, or to some unknown concurrent factors introduced at the same time. However, as a clinical demonstration the data are suggestive and illustrate the potential for the methods in more carefully controlled trials. (See below for discussion of single-subject designs).

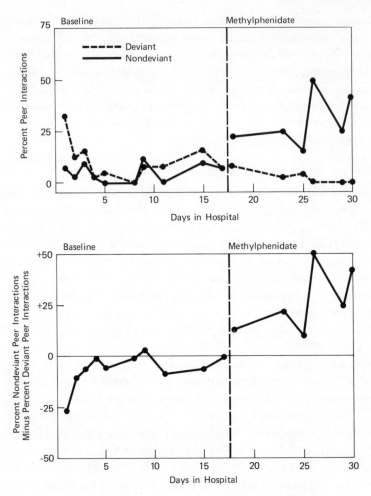

FIGURE 1.   Effects of methylphenidate on peer interactions in aggressive twelve-year-old boy. Peer interactions based upon sixteen minutes direct time-sampling
observation.

Figure 2 shows data on a mute, isolative, and withdrawn ten-year-old girl
thought to be psychotic. The very stable pretreatment baselines for peer interactions and vocalizations strongly suggest that the higher dose of trifluoperazine
has caused greater positive peer interactions and vocalizations, though the variability of the effect is also apparent. These data are noteworthy in that concurrent
ratings by the ward staff failed to detect any drug effect at the time.

The direct methods allow for a much more precise investigation of the relation
between drug and environmental effects. For example, it will be noted that the
large increases in peer interactions occur on days 112, 130, and 137, and this

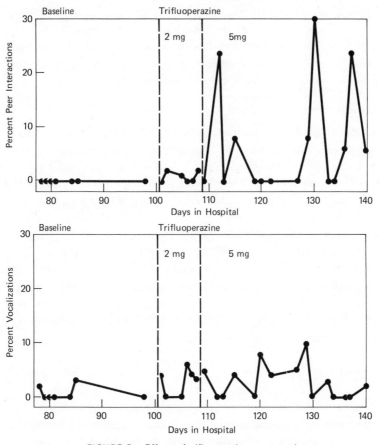

FIGURE 2. Effects of trifluoperazine upon peer interactions and vocalizations in a mute, isolative ten-year-
old girl.

leads to the possibility of determining what specific factors on those days might
be interacting with the drug since the effect is much less apparent on other days.
Visiting days with parents, outings, or other events might be possible "triggers"
for a behavior unavailable to the child prior to medication. As opposed to a general "improvement" rating such data allow for testing hypotheses regarding precisely defined factors that either facilitate or inhibit a generalized drug effect.

Direct behavioral observations also have drawbacks. They depend upon carefully trained observers and the presence of observers may influence the behavior
being observed unless the children are sufficiently adapted to their presence.
Moreover, the techniques are frequently exhausting to the observer over any extended periods of time since very precise limits are usually set with regard to the
recording and timing of observations. A further issue is that discrete behaviors
may sometimes be insensitive to drug effects while more global judgments that

take the whole context into account will pick up the effects. It has frequently been found in adult psychopharmacology that global measures are among the most sensitive indicators, despite their other disadvantages. A recent paper by Werry (1976) provides a complete discussion of issues in the application of direct behavioral methods in pediatric psychopharmacology.

B. Rating Methods in Pediatric Psychopharmacology *

Reference has already been made to the ECDEU rating scales now widely used in drug studies with children. This battery includes a rating scale for psychiatrists, teacher and parent ratings, and a behavior inventory suitable for inpatient drug studies. Discussion of these instruments has appeared in a previous publication (Conners, 1973) and the teacher and parent scales have been standardized on normal populations (Werry, Sprague, and Cohen, 1975) and widely used in drug trials (Kupietz, Bialer, and Winsberg, 1972; Conners, 1972; Sprague, Christensen and Werry, 1974). A short ten-item subscale has proved extremely useful and sensitive in drug trials of hyperkinetic children and has the virtue of being brief enough to allow repeated assessments during a study. This scale shows a high correlation with hyperactivity and conduct disturbance factors from the longer scales (Werry, Sprague, and Cohen, 1975). In this scale the rating items are simply summed to give a total score.

The distinction between a direct observation and a rating or global judgment is not absolute: even direct time-sampling methods require some degree of integrative judgment by assigning a carefully defined behavior to some class (e.g., "hitting," or "on-task"). Virtually no behavior can be said to occur in the absence of coding rules used by the observer. It is frequently assumed that a direct observation (such as time sampling or interval sampling) is more accurate than a judgment made after the fact in which a number of behaviors are subsumed under one trait name by an observer. This is in fact a very knotty problem going to the heart of measurement and epistemology in behavioral science.

One of the major issues has to do with the relevance or meaningfulness of behaviors selected for direct observation. This issue was one of the key problems addressed in Murray's seminal *Explorations in Personality* (1938). Murray noted that:

Some psychologists may prefer to limit themselves to the study of one kind of episode. For instance, they may study the responses of a great number of individuals to a specific situation. They may attempt to discover what changes in the situation bring about important changes in response. But, since every response is partially determined by the after-ef-

* Portions of this section were presented to the FDA Subcommittee on Pediatric Psychopharmacology

fects of previous experiences, the psychologist will never fully understand an episode if he abstracts it from ontogeny, the developmental history of the individual. (p. 2)

Murray eschews limited time samples of behavior because of the difficulty of relating the behavior to a meaningful pattern of which the organism is a part. This issue of the behavior-in-isolation vs. the behavior-in-context is still one that confronts every observer who wishes to abstract from the total flow of behavior those elements that are useful.

The process whereby an observer comes to abstract and synthesize some specific samples of behavior is in fact a somewhat mysterious and unknown matter. It is known, however, that the 'set' of the observer, for example, degree of contact with the subject, language framework, values, are variables influencing the act of observing. In the simplest sense, the ego of the observer influences both what he chooses to look at and how he characterizes what he sees. Moreover the "Heisenberg Principle" of observing applies: most observers are in the process of shaping the behavior they are ostensibly recording or observing, a fact often salient in the parent and teacher observing a child, which is one basis for claiming that such observers have limited value in an 'objective' measurement of behavior.

One of the important landmarks in the measurement of behavior is the *Measurement of Meaning* (Osgood et al. 1957). In his studies Osgood found that an enormous number of adjectives applied to behavior could frequently be reduced to three sources of variance: an evaluative dimension (good-bad), a power dimension (strong-weak), and an activity dimension (fast-slow). This formed the basis for his widely used technique of the semantic differential. The point of those studies in this context is that these categories appear to influence strongly almost all human judgments involving the assignment of a meaning to ongoing samples of behavior; like Kant's use of concepts such as space-time, they appear to form the windows through which reality is observed. Thus, a teacher looking at a child in the classroom uses a strong evaluative dimension: relating the behavior to the rules, to the structure and purposes of the classroom, and to a concept of good-bad in the classroom context (and perhaps elsewhere as well). Parents who judge a child "active" must perforce do so with respect to their own internal standards of what is permissible or desirable, not just to "what is" or "out there."

Behaviorists typically try to minimize factors such as an evaluative frame of reference by carefully defining the rules for classifying a particular motor act, but this is often an ideal rather than a fact. A particular vocalization or motor act will still frequently be characterized by reference to its meaning in a social context (what constitutes "hitting" or "swearing" can be remarkably vague and requires long lists of qualifiers to achieve reliability). The questions one has after such a definition is arrived at, and the behavior appropriately sampled, is "so what?" "Does it matter, does it relate to anything in the real world, is it sensitive to environmental manipulation?" These are empirical questions that may give disappointing answers. For example, Werry (1976) has commented that such direct observational measures can be disappointingly insensitive to drug effects easily detected by global ratings.

One explanation may have to do with the ability of the observer to evaluate the behavior in a context with respect to standards or meanings *supplied by the observer*. Since these are minimized in the direct-observation samples, the latter may be less sensitive to certain interventions; the bits of behavior may be too tiny to catch the relevance of a larger pattern or whole which the observer supplies. Some might argue that this approach leads to a naive subjectivism and away from what is "in the child" or "out there." But again, this appears to be a matter of empirical study, and to date global rating scales often come out much better in terms of utility, sensitivity to environmental changes, and ability to predict other classes of behavior.

The fact seems to be that qualities of a child such as "impulsive" or "distractible" require a sufficiently long sample of behavior in order for these adjectives to be applied by someone who has certain standards of these concepts. "Restlessness" may show very little correlation with actual wiggling, running, fidgeting, etc. because this is a category that observers employ when a certain quality of behavior reaches some threshold, probably a threshold related more to the tolerance of the observer than to some intrinsic property of the child; or it is a quality which is inferred or attributed to the child by matching a sample of behavior against some internal schema of how goal-directed the behavior is rather than its actual quantity. One might argue that such scales are in fact the most meaningful from a behavioral point of view precisely because they abstract behaviors that have social significance.

C. Recent Ratings Scales

Bell, Waldrop, and Weller (1972) describe a rating system appropriate for nursery-school-age children in which characteristics of hyperactivity and withdrawal are rated. As noted in our previous discussion of rating scales (Conners, 1973), a conduct-disturbance dimension and an anxiety-fearfulness dimension have emerged in most studies of a diversity of traits in school-age children. Bell et al.'s scale has eleven points in which categories of frenetic play, induction of intervention, inability to delay, emotional aggression, nomadic play, and spilling-throwing are rated (hyperactivity dimension), and vacant staring, closeness to adult base, and chronic fearfulness are rated for the withdrawal factor. Results are based on observations of nursery school children at least two hours a day, with ratings made on a day-to-day basis or at the end of a month. Home visits were made to develop some of the ratings. The ratings were also summarized on a weekly basis in one of the studies. A factor scoring system based on normative data is provided from which one may compute a total hyperactivity and total withdrawal score and compare it with the optimal cutoff point for differentiating the normal from extreme cases. Although no comparisons with clinically diagnosed samples have been made, and no drug studies carried out, this instrument should prove to be extremely useful in selecting subjects in the kindergarten or nursery-school period for investigative studies. Reliabilities of the individual items is quite good, ranging from .59 to .94. The provision of a simple factor scoring system should also make the instrument useful for following children over time and detecting changes due to intervention.

Blunden, Spring, and Greenberg (1974) carried out an extensive validation of their Classroom Behavior Inventory (CBI) using 320 kindergarten boys. The scale uses ten categories of behavior associated with the hyperkinetic syndrome (restlessness, impulsivity, distractibility, low concentration, low perseverance, irritability, resentfulness, cheerfulness, social participation, and verbal expression), with four items in each category rated on a four-point scale ("not at all like the child" to "very much like the child"). Four factors emerged from a factor analysis computation: Factor I, labeled Hyperactivity, included items from the restlessness, impulsivity, distractibility, low concentration, and low perseverance categories; Factor II (Hostility) included the irritability and resentfulness categories; Factor III (Sociability) included cheerfulness, social participation, and verbal expression items; and Factor IV, accounting for only 3 percent of the variance, was considered uninterpretable.

Concurrent validity was measured by comparing the CBI with direct time sampling in the classroom utilizing fifteen-second intervals over a fifteen-minute period three times for a week. Thus, each subject had forty-five minutes of direct observation. Interobserver agreement ranged from 71 percent to 78 percent, calculated by determining the ratio of the number of fifteen-second intervals in which the selected behavior was observed by both observers to the number of fifteen-second intervals in which the behavior was observed by at least one observer (this method is subject to spurious inflation as noted in Werry's chapter, 1976).

The results were striking: only one of the CBI scales (impulsiveness) was actually significantly correlated with its direct observation counterpart ($r = .50$). Of the forty-nine correlations in the matrix, only nine were actually significant, with six of those being correlations of the direct observations with teacher's ratings of impulsiveness. Teachers made global judgments of whether the children had behavior disorders or not, and on eight of ten teacher ratings there were significant differences while only one of the direct observation scores differentiated the two groups (impulsiveness).

The authors suggest that either the low stability of the directly observed behaviors from the forty-five-minute sample, or limited inter-teacher reliabilities may have attenuated the correspondence of the two data sets. They also suggest that the teachers may have been using essentially only one "real" dimension, impulsiveness. However, one might equally well argue that the teachers' ratings were valid, and the directly observed behaviors invalid due to their highly context-specific, unrepresentative nature. Greenberg et al. (1972) have shown that the CBI is somewhat sensitive to drug effects, but once again we are left to wonder what is really being measured.

Davids (1971) has provided a clinical rating instrument for hyperkinesis which uses seven items rated on a six-point scale. The instrument was published with full awareness that reliability and validity had not been established. It was used in a study comparing Dexedrine and placebo by Denhoff, Davids, and Hawkins (1971). Three of the items (activity, short attention span, and impulsiveness) discriminated at a significant level between drug and placebo. Drug effects were prominent in those children whose teachers gave a rating of four or more on each of the six scales. Neither drug effects nor correlations with teacher scales were significant in the parent ratings using the same form.

The Children's Pathology Index (CPI) (Alderton and Hoddinott, 1968) is a scale for inpatient observation of children that has received careful study. The ranking of descriptive statements from "best" (5) to worst (1) was verified by using six trained judges and computing coefficients of concordance, which ranged from 1.0 to .67, with twenty-two reaching 0.9 or better and all but five 0.8 or better. A factor analysis of the instrument produced four factors. The four factors, disturbed behavior toward adults, neurotic constriction, destructive behavior, and disturbed self-perception, appear to be similar to dimensions found on several other instruments. In particular, the conduct-disorder and anxiety factors seem to be constant dimensions of most instruments.

Reliabilities were computed using four raters, twenty-eight days apart and forty-two days apart. The twenty-eight-day reliabilities were .85, .40, .79, and .79 for the four factors respectively; the forty-two-day reliabilities were .75, .72, .79, and .88.

Concurrent validity was investigated by comparing time samples of aggressive behavior with the Factor 1 scores. A correlation of .59 was obtained. A biserial correlation of .82 was obtained between Factor 1 scores and psychiatrists' discharge prognosis for community adjustment. This means, of course, that the psychiatrist simply felt that more aggressive children would adjust more poorly. The actual patient status at eighteen months after discharge was significantly associated with all four factors, utilizing categories of institutionalized, remaining in the community and remaining in the community without significant difficulty. To what extent these findings reflect the self-fulfilling prophecy of the psychiatric discharge prognosis and recommendation is unclear. But it is notable that most of the effects are accounted for by the difference between the hospitalized and the nonhospitalized children—a result compatible with this hypothesis. If the psychiatrist both made a prognosis and assigned the children to other institutions, this would not reflect true independent predictive validity of the instrument. A further study showed that the CPI did not show significant inter-institutional profile differences in a comparison of four similar institutions. While this finding may imply the "universality" of the instrument as suggested by the authors, it could also be due to insensitivity.

The Deviant Behavior Inventory (DBI) is an instrument intensively studied by Novick et al. (1966) and currently in use by this writer as a screening device for parents of children admitted to an inpatient unit. The value of the instrument is in its careful wording of items (readability), its completeness (237 items), its Q-sort administration, the use of a "not sure" category, a clearly specified time reference, a procedure for self-correction of endorsements by partial resorting, and a focussed inquiry to document endorsed deviant behaviors. A careful look at the procedure of this study has much to recommend it for those who rely too cavalierly on parent-administered forms of this type.

Specifically, the authors found that parents failed to pick as "True" a substantial number of items known from independent sources to be present; and conversely, that of those items picked as "True," a substantial proportion were ultimately judged to be invalid. Despite its limitations, this type of instrument serves a useful screening function by covering virtually all areas of symptomatology of relevance to the eight- to twelve-year-old age range, and if administered carefully can provide detailed parent descriptions useful in the evaluation of therapy or in follow-up. It is an instrument too long for frequent or repeated use, but the selection of *target* symptoms could be a useful way of generating an individualized scale of moderate length for each patient.

Another method for inpatient observations has been provided in the Children's Behavior Inventory (CBI) (Burdock and Hardesty, 1964). This scale utilizes concrete behavioral events arranged according to the chronological age at which they are considered deviant. Although the behavioral events are quite specific, they are recorded *after* the behavior has occurred over some specified time period, thus making it feasible for nurses or other ward staff to use after the behavior has occurred, at some time convenient for recording. Although little has been published regarding its use in drug trials, it is possible to achieve good reliabilities with minimal training. The instrument appears to be drug sensitive, as illustrated in Figures 3 and 4, which show scores (grouped according to a priori categories) for the day and evening shifts in a pediatric psychiatric inpatient unit. The rating were made by nurses twice daily for the half hours before lunch and dinner, and for the half hour during lunch and dinner.

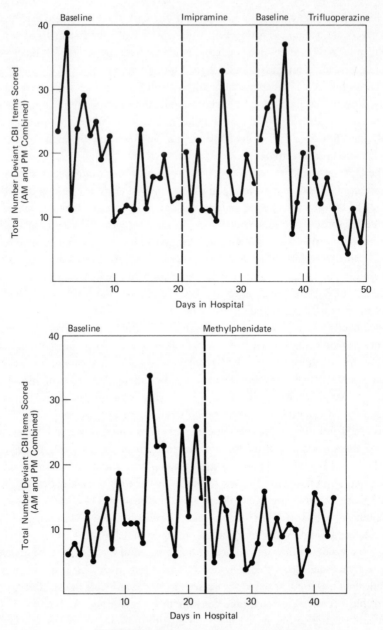

FIGURES 3 and 4. Drug effects upon behavioral observations made by child care staff (data combines
two one-half hour samples from morning and evening).

This type of scale combines the best features of direct observation (specificity of behavior, reliability, limited time of observation) with those of more global rating scales (sensitivity, ease of training, flexibility, molar segments of behavior). The main point to be made with both the direct and global methods of assessment is that such methods provide quantitative, reliable, and sensitive measures for drug studies with children. The usefulness, empirical validity, and theoretical value of such instruments is of course a complex matter, but in the present state of the art these methods provide useful examples of alternative methods for psychopharmacologic investigations with children.

Whether these or other instruments are used, certain principles of scale construction should be followed in selecting or devising instruments for assessing change attributable to medication (as well as changes attributed to other treatments or nonspecific factors such as placebo effects). 1. The reliability of the instrument should be demonstrated *over the time periods to be used in a drug trial*. Technical issues of establishing reliability may be found in Hawkins and Dotson (1975) and in *The Handbook of Psychiatric Rating Scales* (DHEW, undated). 2. The scales should measure states rather than traits; i.e., the characteristics must show some normal variability upon repeated measurements rather than reflect stable personality or dispositional characteristics not likely to change over the time course of the drug trial. 3. The scales should show sensitivity to treatment, preferably demonstrated sensitivity to drugs. 4. The scales should cover the range of symptoms or target behaviors supposed to be influenced by the drug. In general, scales which measure existing deviant behavior are likely to be more sensitive than scales which measure deficit behaviors that have not made an appearance in the child's behavioral repertoire.

D. Performance and Laboratory Measures

Virtually any standardized laboratory or performance test is feasible as a measure of change attributable to drugs. A number of such measures have been used in pediatric drug research, including intelligence tests, school achievement tests, motor development scales, paired-associate learning, continuous performance tests, seat activity, recognition learning and memory, flicker fusion, reaction time, EEG, psychophysiologic measures such as galvanic skin response or finger blood volume, and many more. Issues in the use of such measures have been discussed by Sprague (1973). In general such measures cannot stand by themselves in tests of drug efficacy since they must always be related to the relevant molar and life situations for which drug therapy is indicated. But they can ensure that sensitive measures are available to detect drug effects not noted by less precise observational procedures, and they are essential in testing specific hypotheses regarding the mode of action of drugs at a behavioral level. Thus, for example, if a drug is thought to impair concentration or speed of reaction, a continuous performance or reaction-time method is preferable to simple global estimates or even direct observation. The latter may be too insensitive to pick up fine increments or decrements in performance attributable to a centrally acting drug. Moreover, such measures are easily compared from one study to another and can be interpreted in terms of the standardization data often available for such instruments. In general, a combination of both objective and indirect methods of observation are useful in documenting drug efficacy and safety.

E. Neuro-developmental measures

It is almost always desirable in drug research with children to assess the neurological integrity of the child prior to any drug therapy. Apart from standard medical neurological examinations before, during, and after the drug trials, subtle changes in coordination, rhythm, balance, posture, and sensory-motor integration may be expected to affect the outcome of drug treatment as well as to vary because of drug treatment—either as a performance improvement or side effect or toxic reaction to the treatment itself. The difficulty with most informal procedures is that they have been insufficiently standardized on normal children. Such methods are essentially behavioral assessments and should conform to the basic principles of standardization, including reliability and appropriate comparison norms, that are expected of other psychological test functions.

One such standardized (though inadequately normed) instrument is the soft sign neurological examination developed by Close (1973) and used in the ECDEU battery. This measure has the advantage of being usable by a clinician without elaborate equipment and has a careful instructional manual and quantified performance measures (e.g., rather than simply indicating that a child passed or failed the test for stereognosis, the examiner awards one point for each of two recognition trials, a third point if the object is recognized only when seen, and a fourth point if the child is unable to pick the object out of a box with other items).

Another measure successfully used in drug trials with children is the Lincoln-Oseretsky Motor Development Scale, as modified by Sloan (1955). In many respects such a method has much to recommend it over the "soft sign" procedures used by most clinicians. The test is somewhat lengthy, but a recent modified version (Bialer et al., 1975) has been shortened and standardized for use in drug studies. It provides factors which can measure specific motor processes, covers a broad range of neuro-integrative functions, is reliable and allows developmental comparisons with normal children.

F. Projective and Other Measures

It is sometimes desirable to assess the impact of drugs upon a child's affective responsiveness, perceptual style, or other functions not easily defined by direct observation or ratings. The Holtzman Inkblot Test (1961) has been successfully used to measure diagnostic and treatment effects in a drug study with children (Conners, 1965). This test, like the Rorschach, utilizes inkblots, but uses only one response per card, and contains two forty-five-card sets carefully standardized for repeated testing. A wide variety of validity studies suggests that important features of childhood psychopathology may be measured by the instrument (Hill, 1972), and the psychometric sophistication of the instrument has much to recommend it, especially for testing specific hypotheses regarding drug effects.

This author has used a number of scoring systems applied to the Thematic Apperception Test (Murray, 1943), but has never found a single drug effect on such measures.

Perceptual style measures, such as the Children's Embedded Figures Test, and the Matching Familiar Figures Test have been successfully used in studies of the hyperkinetic child, both differentiating such children from normal children (Douglas, 1974), and showing drug-treatment effects (Campbell, 1974; Campbell, Douglas, and Morgenstern, 1971). Such measures can be useful if traits of impulsivity, reflectivity, and perceptual field articulation are hypothesized as drug effects or areas of function thought to be impaired in the sample studied.

There are important methodological issues to deal with whenever a battery of tests such as mentioned above are used as dependent variables in a drug study.

TABLE 1

Most Frequently Used Tests and Percent of Subtest Variables Reported Showing Significant Change with Drug

Test	Times Used	Variables Per Test	Variables Total	Significant No. of Times	Significant Percent
Bender-Gestalt	11	1	11	2	18
WISC	10	13	130	6	5
Draw-a-Person	8	1	8	3	38
Frostig	7	6	42	6	14
Porteus Maze T.O.	6	1	6	4	66
Lincoln-Oseretsky	6	3	18	2	11
WRAT	6	3	18	3	17
Graduated Holes	4	4	16	4	25
Paired Associates	4	2	8	3	38
Continuous Performance	4	2	8	2	25
Reaction Time	4	1	4	2	50

Data from Knights (1974).

Many tests contribute multiple scores and it is often desirable to examine the pattern of subscore changes, such as on the Wechsler scales. However, one should remember that such subscales are often unreliable and that *change* scores are even more unreliable.

Moreover, a few tests with several subscales pose a problem in statistical interpretation since one may expect a certain number of significant changes due to chance alone. This issue has been discussed by Knights (1974). Table 1 shows tests most frequently used and the percent showing significant drug effects in eighteen studies with children. Table 2 presents various test measures grouped according to major category of function, the number of times used in eighteen studies, and the number and percent of significant drug effects. Although these tables provide a rough guide to the sensitivity of certain instruments, they also show that one must be cautious about the total number of significance tests performed in a drug study since many such measures will allow for a capitalization on chance. One method recommended if the number of study subjects is sufficiently large is a multivariate analysis of variance (MANOVA) which can test for overall drug effect before examining individual contrasts between drug and placebo groups for several different test measures.

TABLE 2

Total Number of Subtests Used in 18 Studies Grouped by Type of Test

		Variables	
Ability and Tests	Total	No. Significant	Percent Significant
1. Motility:	5	2	40
Stabilimetric chair			
Actometer			
Tremorgraph			
Motor Activity			
Distance moved			
Percent time moving			
2. Complex motor:	9	3	33
Maze			
Holes			
Pegboard			
Motor coordination			
Lincoln-Oseretsky			
Motor inhibition			
3. Attention and vigilance:	36	8	31
Continuous performance test			
Picture completion			
Porteus maze			
Embedded figures			
Visual discrimination			

TABLE 2 (continued)

Ability and Tests	Variables		
	Total	No. Significant	Percent Significant
4. New learning: Paired associations Matching familiar figures Discrimination learning Digit symbol	13	4	31
5. Intelligence measures: WISC FS I.Q. Performance I.Q. Verbal I.Q. Primary mental abilities	33	10	30
6. Visual-motor, spatial: Bender-Gestalt Draw-a-Person Frostig Spatial orientation	62	18	29

7. Auditory perception and memory:
Auditory-discrimination
    memory
    synthesis
Speech noise
Visual-auditory memory
Digit span
	24	6	25

8. Verbal fluency: Fluency Naming animals and colors Tell a story	20	5	25
9. Simple motor: Tapping speed Reaction time	31	3	23
10. Language learning and achievement: Information Comprehension Vocabulary Similarities WRAT Reading speed comprehension	68	7	10
11. Problem solving: Picture arrangement Block design Object assembly Coding Arithmetic	50	1	2

Data from Knights (1974).

G. Measurement of Side Effects and Toxicity

Children may show side effects of drug treatment that differ from those that adults show. They may not be able to recognize or inform the physician reliably of drug-induced symptoms. Therefore, methods of assessment for side effects are different for children and adults. Little attention has been given to this issue in childhood psychopharmacology, but a first step has been taken in the collaborative efforts under the auspices of the ECDEU. Separate side-effects checklists for parents, physician, and self-report have been developed (Goffman, 1973), but these measures have not yet received study as measuring instruments per se. Nevertheless, certain principles should be mentioned: first, the assessment should include measures taken before treatment, since many complaints of children are transient and unrelated to treatment; second, judgments from several sources should be considered. The teacher may be the best observer for side effects relating to the child's academic and social functioning, while the parent may be more valid as an observer of neuro-vegetative changes such as eating and sleeping. Responses such as "dry mouth" or "blurred vision" may be more appropriate for direct observation in the clinical setting than by self-report or other methods. It is surprising that so little attention has been given to this important problem and that these assessments are often relegated to scanty and informal methods in drug studies with children.

Many complexities surround the measurement of toxicity in drug research with children. Among these are differences in protein-binding at different ages, the development of liver function, and differences in metabolism for a wide variety of chemical substances at different ages. Gershon (1973) makes the important point that widely quoted "normal values" of laboratory measures for children are not infrequently based upon a small number of subjects of diverse ages. A large source of uncertainty comes from the variability of laboratory standards. In a recent study, this author found that over 15 percent of the values taken on children prior to treatment were abnormal, but upon repeat testing all such abnormalities vanished! Without a pretreatment repeated baseline, such results could confound any true assessment of the toxicity of a particular treatment.

DESIGN AND STATISTICAL ISSUES

In principle a drug study is a straightforward experimental design in which the drug is the independent variable and the various symptoms, measures, or functions of the child are the dependent variables. Randomization of subjects, control groups, placebo, double-blind methods, and the like are too well known to warrant comment. However, because of practical, ethical, or logistic issues many studies cannot meet the ideal requirements sought in controlled scientific investigations. If matching of subjects in experimental and control groups is not feasible, or if the number of subjects for a particular diagnosis is small—as is likely in studies of severe conditions such as childhood autism—consideration should be given to within-subject or even single-subject designs, a methodology frequently used in behavioral research and only recently beginning to appear in psychopharmacologic investigations. Werry (1970) has summarized a number of within-subject drug studies with children.

Although such designs present many important advantages, such as the reduction of between-subject variability (which is usually the largest source of variance in any behavioral experiment), carry-over effects, and sequence effects, interactions of treatments with order of testing make crossover experiments hazardous. A thorough discussion of such matters is beyond the scope of this chapter, but the reader is referred to the excellent discussions of these and related issues in Levine, Schiele, and Bouthilet (1971).

One common issue worth considering is the problem of statistical analysis in drug trials. Usually the experiment will consist of a treatment group and one or more control groups, with measures before and after treatment. These measures will be either categorical data or dimensional data for which chi-square or parametric statistics, respectively, may be indicated. The mistake is sometimes made of treating repeated measures on categorical data as though they were measures from independent subjects, thus inflating the N (number) for the chi-square analysis. Fisher (1962) has described this problem in the context of drug studies, remedied by the use of a repeated measure chi-square as described by McNemar (1955). In a recent publication Klein et al. (1975) has provided a thoughtful discussion of the issues surrounding parametric analyses on repeated measures in drug studies.

INDEPENDENT VARIABLES IN DRUG RESEARCH

Naturally a drug or other treatments (or controls) constitutes the essential independent variable in most drug research. General principles of experimental design suggest that several variations of the independent variable (e.g., several dosage levels of the drug) provide a more powerful manipulation of the independent variable than a single level of treatment. Thus, when possible it is desirable to examine dose-response functions in order to ascertain optimal therapeutic levels, the dosage at which side effects or toxicity occur, and which functions are affected at different dose levels. With children, however, great individual variability in response is the rule, which means that many drug trials will consist of finding the optimal level before assessing therapeutic effects on certain behavioral or physiological response systems. The latter method is usually preferred in comparisons of separate (between-subjects) treatment groups, while the examination of dose-response curves is more appropriate for within-subject designs where the large inter-individual differences do not obscure dose-response relationships.

Heterogeneity of subject populations is the most significant problem in conducting drug research from the point of view of the total contribution to the variance of the experiment. In order to minimize such factors it is sometimes desirable to utilize different diagnoses, personality traits, physiological parameters, etc. as independent variables in addition to the drug treatment, thus allowing one to examine drug-by-patient-characteristic interactions. For example, high and low arousal subjects, hyperkinetics and neurotics, severe vs. mild disorders, etc., can serve as additional independent variables, usually by splitting the drug treatment and placebo treatments within a category in a factorial design. An example is the study of the pharmacokinetics of amphetamine in brain-damaged and nondamaged hyperkinetics by Epstein, et al. (1968) in which differences in urinary excretion of amphetamine were found to be different for the two groups, with different effects related to pH and different side effects due to the treatment.

Control over the drug as the independent variable requires a thorough documentation system which records changes in dosage levels, duration of treatment, unanticipated stopping of drug, compliance, concurrent medications, and intercurrent illnesses which might affect the interpretation of results. Naturally, such information will have to be carefully related to behavioral and other data reflecting drug response.

ETHICAL ISSUES IN DRUG RESEARCH WITH CHILDREN

The oldest guideline regarding medical treatments is the physician's injunction: "First, do no harm." Arnold (1975), a pediatric pharmacologic investigator, has also added the injunction: "Second, do not withhold good treatment." These two injunctions taken together imply that any drug used should have thorough animal, as well as phase I and phase II studies on adults before investigation with children; that the drug should offer some advantage over other available treatments; and that the benefit though likely, should be in some doubt. Otherwise straightforward clinical management rather than a study would be justified.

A recurrent issue involving informed consent concerns the use and instructions regarding placebo effects. The ethical dilemma is the concern that telling the patient or guardian that the patient will receive a placebo will vitiate the value of the placebo and bias the outcome of treatment. This is an empirical question with very few data, although one study reports that informing patients ahead of time that they are receiving a placebo does not impair the placebo effect (Park and Covi, 1965). Our own practice has been to inform parents and children that a placebo is being used, that the patient has an equal chance of being assigned to it, but will have the option to receive the other treatment(s) at any time during the study when it is felt that failure to improve warrants it, and that the use of a placebo actually helps confirm the value, if any, of the drug treatment. This latter point can be more forcefully applied for within-subject designs, where the comparison of the child's performance on both the active and inactive agent actually clarifies how much the active agent does *for the particular patient*. Thus, the benefit is not for the sake of children in general, or even "hyperkinetic" or "autistic" children, but the particular individual patient.

That benefit should outweigh the risks of treatment is in general too vague a guideline to employ since seldom are appropriate standards available. It may be impossible, for example, to determine whether the risk of a tardive dyskinesia from a phenothiazine outweighs the benefits to the child and his family of, say, controlling severely agitated behavior in a grossly psychotic youngster. Naturally, common sense indicates that a full explication to the parent and the child of both the risks and the benefits of treatment in a controlled study should always be given, and is generally required by most states and most human-rights review committees. The difficulties come, however, around such issues as the child's autonomy, intelligence, and ability to understand what is in his own best interest. Recent years have seen a steady escalation of the debate between human rights advocates and medical researchers over the limits of responsibility in children and their parents. Thoughtful discussants of these issues (Curran and Beecher, 1969; Beyer, 1975; National Commission for the Protection of Human Subjects in Biomedical and Behavioral Research, 1975, unpublished) have presented views which try to balance the needs of the individual within a research and treatment process against the needs and rights of individual children. Several statements by the Food and Drug Administration and the Department of Health, Education, and Welfare in recent years have responded to this increased concern and awareness, and should be consulted in cases of drug research with children which pose difficult ethical and legal issues (DHEW, 1973; DHEW, 1971). Beecher's comprehensive treatise presents the views of an experienced researcher and scientist covering much of the historical background (Beecher, 1970).

It is common opinion that other treatments should be tried before resorting to drug treatments, but this opinion is often based upon the untested assumption that the other treatments (such as behavior therapy, environmental restructuring, special education) are effective in treating the presenting problems. In fact, very few careful comparative studies of different treatments with children which meet scientific criteria have been carried out. One still has the dilemma that abjuring drug therapy for the sake of a treatment which may cost time and be worthless to boot, has to be considered a risk for the child. Where possible, therefore, such comparative studies of alternative treatments need to be done with the population under study, and as rigorously evaluated as the drug treatment itself.

SUMMARY

This chapter stresses an approach to childhood psychopharmacology which regards subject selection, measurement of independent and dependent variables, and experimental design problems as aspects of scientific research requiring solutions specific to the pediatric age group. Good drug research requires careful operational specification of the target population, defined by rigorous criteria, as well as specification of target symptoms or functions in a replicable, explicit manner. Diagnosis, though basically judgmental and integrative is viewed as a useful and necessary process in which specific criteria for a diagnosis are made operational by ratings or other data sources explicitly tied to the diagnosis. A diagnosis of childhood schizophrenia, for example, is of no value in a drug study unless the specific inclusion and exclusion criteria are set forth, and the manner in which these criteria are used is made clear.

Measurement in childhood psychopharmacology relies on direct observations, teacher and parent ratings, performance tests, and direct examination of the child. Various available instruments for inpatient and outpatient populations are described. These instruments are useful tools in the research process but inevitably leave many issues unresolved, such as the extent to which direct, presumably "objective" data sources are useful as compared with ratings and indirect measures such as performance or laboratory measures. It is suggested that adequate drug studies will generally use multiple points of observation and that no one class or type of method of measurement will suffice. Certain design and statistical issues are mentioned as problems requiring careful attention, and ethical issues specific to children are discussed.

References

Alderton, H., and Hoddinott, B. (1968), The children's pathology index. *Canad. Psychiat. Assn. J.,* *13,* 353–361.

American Academy of Pediatrics. (1975), *Guidelines for evaluation of psychoactive drugs in infants and children.*

APA. *Diagnostics and statistical manual,* 2nd Ed. (DSM-II). Washington, D.C., 1968.

Arnold, L. E. (1975), A humanistic approach to neurochemical research in children. In E. J. Anthony (Ed.), *Explorations in child psychiatry.* New York: Plenum.

Beecher, H. K. (1970), *Research and the individual.* Boston: Little, Brown and Co.

Bell, R., Waldrop, M., and Weller, G. (1972), A rating system for the assessment of hyperactive and withdrawn children in preschool samples. *Am. J. Orthopsychiat., 42,* 23–34.

Beyer, H. A. (1975), The child's right to refuse mental health treatment. *Psychiat. Ann., 15,* 77–90.

Bialer, I., Doll, L., and Winsberg, B. G. (1975), A modified Lincoln-Oseretsky motor development scale: provisional standardization. *Percept. Mot. Skills, 38,* 599–614.

Blunden, D., Spring, C., and Greenberg, L., (1974), Validation of the classroom behavior inventory. *J. Cons. and Clin. Psych., 42,* 84–88.

Burdock, E. L., and Hardesty, A. S. (1964), A children's behavior diagnostic inventory. *Ann. N.Y. Acad. Sci., 105,* 890–896.

Campbell, S. B. (1974) Cognitive styles and behavior problems of clinic boys: A comparison of epileptic, hyperactive, learning-disabled and normal groups. *J. Abnorm. Ch. Psych., 2,* 307–312.

Campbell, S., Douglas, V. I., and Morgenstern, G. (1971), Cognitive styles in hyperactive children and the effect of methylphenidate. *J. Ch. Psych. Psychiat., 12,* 55–67.

Close, J. (1973), Scored neurological examination. *Psychopharmacology Bulletin.* Special Issue, Pharmacotherapy of children. NIMH, pp. 142–150. DHEW Publication No. (HSM) 73–9002.

Conners, C. K. (1965), Effects of brief psychotherapy, drugs and type of disturbance on Holtzman Inkblot Scores in Children. Proceedings of the 73rd Annual Convention of the American Psychological Association, pp. 201–202.

Conners, C. K. (1972), Pharmacotherapy of psychopathology in children. In H. C. Quay and J. S. Werry (Eds.), *Psychopathological disorders of childhood.* New York: John Wiley & Sons, pp. 316–348.

Conners, C. K. (1973), Rating scales for use in drug studies with children. *Psychopharmacology Bull.* Special Issue, Pharmacotherapy of children. NIMH, pp. 9–11.

Curran, W. J., and Beecher, H. K. (1969), Experimentation in children; a reexamination of legal ethical principles. *J.A.M.A., 10,* 77–83.

Davids, A. (1971), An objective instrument for assessing hyperkinesis in children. *J. Learn. Disabil., 4,* 35–37.

Denhoff, E., Davids, A., and Hawkins, A. (1971), Effects of dextroamphetamine on hyperkinetic children; a controlled double blind study. *J. Learn. Disabil., 4,* 27–34.

DHEW (PHS Publication No. 1495). *Handbook of psychiatric rating scales.*

DHEW (1973), *Protection of human subjects.* Proposed policy, 39, *Fed. Reg.* 31742, November 16.

DHEW (1971), *The institutional guide of DHEW policy on protection of human subjects,* DHEW Publication No. (NIH) 72–102, December.

DHEW (1974), *Protection of human subjects.* 45 CFR 46, Sec 46.3(b) 39, *Fed. Reg.* 18917, May.

Doke, L. A. (1976), Assessing children's behavioral deficits. In M. Hersen and A. S. Bellack (Eds.), *Behavioral assessment: A practical handbook.* New York: Pergamon Press.

Douglas, V. (1974), Differences between normal and hyperkinetic children. In C. K. Conners (Ed.), *Clinical use of stimulant drugs in children,* Amsterdam: Excerpta Medica.

Epstein, L. C., Lasagna, L., Conners, C. K., and Rodriques, A. (1968), Correlation of dextroamphetamine excretion and drug response in hyperkinetic children. *J. Nerv. Ment. Dis., 146,* 136–146.

Fish, B., and Shapiro, T. (1965), A typology of children's psychiatric disorders, I: Its application to a controlled evaluation of treatment. *J. Am. Acad. Ch. Psychiat., 4,* 32–52.

Fisher, S. (1962), Use of chi-square in simple crossover designs. *Brit. J. Psychiat., 108,* 406–410.

Gershon, S. (1973), Pediatric psychopharmacology—clinical laboratory standards. *Psychopharmacology Bull.* Special Issue, Pharmacotherapy of children. NIMH, pp. 167–181.

Goffman, H. (1973), Interval and final rating sheets on side effects. *Psychopharm. Bull.* Special Issue, Pharmacotherapy of children. NIMH, pp. 182–186.

Greenberg, L., Deem, M. A., and McMahon, S. (1972), Effects of dextroamphetamine, chlorpromazine, and hydroxyzine on behavior and performance in hyperactive children. *Amer. J. of Psychiat., 129,* 532–539.

Group for Advancement of Psychiatry (1966), *Psychopathological disorders in childhood: Theoretical considerations and a proposed classification.* Vol. VI, Report No. 62, June.

Hawkins, R., and Dotson, V. (1975), Reliability scores that delude; an Alice in Wonderland trip through the misleading characteristics of interobserver agreement scores in interval recording. In E. Ramp and G. Semb (Eds.), *Behavior analysis: Areas of research and application.* Englewood Cliffs, N.J.: Prentice-Hall, pp. 359–376.

Hill, E. (1972), *The Holtzman inkblot technique.* San Francisco: Jossey-Bass.

Holtzman, W. H. (1961), *Guide to administration and scoring: Holtzman inkblot technique.* New York: Psychological Corp.

Klein, D., and Gittelman-Klein, R. (1974), Diagnosis of minimal brain dysfunction and hyperkinetic syndrome. In C. K. Conners (Ed.), *Clinical use of stimulant drugs in children,* Amsterdam: Excerpta Medica.

Klein, D. F., Ross, D. C., and Feldman, S. (1975), Analysis and display of psychopharmacological data. *J. Psychiat. Res., 12,* 125–147.

Knights, R. M. (1973), Problems of criteria in diagnosis: A profile similarity approach. In *Minimal brain dysfunction. Ann. N.Y. Acad. Sci., 205,* 124–131.

Knights, R. M. (1974), Psychometric assessment of stimulant induced behavior change. In C. K. Conners (Ed.), *Clinical use of stimulant drugs in children,* Amsterdam: Excerpta Medica.

Kupietz, S., Bialer, I., and Winsberg, B. (1972), A behavior rating scale for assessing improvement in behaviorally deviant children: a preliminary investigation. *Am. J. Psychiat., 128,* 1432–1436.

Levine, J., Schiele, B. C., and Bouthilet, L. (Eds.), (1971), *Principles and problems in establishing the efficacy of psychotropic agents.* PHS Publication No. 2138.

Lipman, R. S. (1974), NIMH-PRB support of research in minimal brain dysfunction in children. In C. K. Conners (Ed.), *Clinical use of stimulant drugs in children.* Amsterdam: Excerpta Medica.

Mann, R. A. (1976), Behavioral excesses in children, In M. Hersen and A. S. Bellack (Eds.), *Behavioral assessment: A practical handbook.* New York: Pergamon Press.

McNemar, Q. (1955), *Psychological statistics,* 2nd Ed. New York: John Wiley and Sons, pp. 57–61.

Monkman, M. (1972), *A milieu therapy program for behaviorally disturbed children.* Springfield: Charles C. Thomas.

Murray, H. A. (1938), *Explorations in personality.* New York: Oxford Univ. Press.

Murray, H. A. (1943), *The thematic apperception test manual.* Cambridge: Harvard Univ. Press.

National Commission for the Protection of Human Subjects in Biomedical and Behavioral Research. (1975), Children and the mentally disabled as research subjects, Unpublished.

NIMH (undated): *The documentation of clinical psychotropic drug trials.* T. McGlashon (Ed.).

Novick, J., Rosenfield, E., Bloch, D. a., and Dawson, D. (1966), Ascertaining deviant behavior in children. *J. Consult. Psych., 30* 230–238.

Osgood, C. E., Suci, G. J., and Tannenbaum, P. H. (1957), *The measurement of meaning.* Urbana: Univ. of Ill. Press.

Park, L., and Covi, L. (1965), Nonblind placebo trial. *Arch. Gen. Psychiat., 12,* 336–345.

Rutter, M., and Graham, P. (1968), The reliability and validity of psychiatric assessment of the child, I: Interview with the child. *Brit. J. Psychiat., 114,* 653–659.

Rutter, M., Levbovici, S., Eisenberg, L., Sneznevskij, A., Sadoun, R., Brooke, E., and Lin, T. (1969), A tri-axial classification of mental disorders in childhood. *J. Ch. Psych. & Psychiatr., 10,* 41–61.

Sloan, W. (1955), The Lincoln-Oseretsky motor development scale. *Genetic Psychol. Monogr., 51,* 183–252.

Sprague, R. L. (1973), Recommended performance measures for Psychotropic drug investigations. *Psychopharmacology Bull.* Special Issue, Pharmacotherapy of children. NIMH, pp. 85–88.

Sprague, R. L., Christensen, D. E., and Werry, J. S. (1974), Experimental psychology and stimulant drugs. In C. K. Conners (Ed.), *Clinical use of stimulant drugs in children.* Amsterdam: Excerpta Medica.

Werry, J. S. (1970), Some clinical and laboratory studies of psychotropic drugs in children: An overview. In W. L. Smith (Ed.), *Drugs and cerebral function.* Springfield: Charles C. Thomas.

Werry, J. S. (1973), Diagnosis for psychopharmacological studies in children. In *Psychophar-macology Bull.* Special Issue, Pharmacotherapy of children, NIMH, pp. 89–96.

Werry, J. (1976), Behavior observations and activity measures for use in pediatric psychophar-macology. U.S. Food and Drug Administration, (Subcommittee on Pediatric Psychophar-macology).

Werry, J. S., Sprague, R. L., and Cohen, M. (1975), Conners' teacher rating scale for use in drug studies with children—an empirical study. *J. Abnorm. Ch. Psych.*, *3*, 217–229.

Chapter Four

DEVELOPMENTAL CONSIDERATIONS IN PSYCHOPHARMACOLOGY: THE INTERACTION OF DRUGS AND DEVELOPMENT

Theodore Shapiro, M.D.

DEFINITION OF A PROBLEM

Child psychiatrists use pharmacological agents in order to affect behavior. Insofar as the behavior to be affected occurs in a growing and changing organism, the medication can be said to influence developmental patterning. Most child psychiatrists consider themselves practitioners of developmental psychiatry suited by their training to deal with the interplay of drugs with changing behavior. However, they would be unhappy with the notion of "controlling" behavior. Similarly, concepts such as "inhibiting" and "disinhibiting" sound too neurophysiological and mechanistically gruff in a human setting. The notion of "modulating" behavior in order to encourage a new adaptive state or phase might be more salutary.

These preliminary comments are made to highlight the problem the child psychiatrist has in accepting an appropriate framework for the use of medication for children. Stated in this form it is a problem that requires the integration of language of disciplines learned during medical training with the language of developmental propositions that has become the major scaffolding of child psychiatry. This is not so easy a task since it is clear that when we use pharmacological agents, we are attempting to change some substrate and have therefore tacitly accepted a mechanistic contribution to the emergence of behavior. To use, then, only dynamic terminology makes it difficult to include the contributions made to developmental psychology from other sources.

How can we extricate ourselves from the paradox that a group of clinicians devoted to the well-being of children, humanistically oriented, and geared towards developmental principles will avoid or discourage the use of medication, because doing so applies itself to a level of organization that implies firm brain-behavior correlation?

Perhaps the antagonism is a pseudo-conflict! Bastardized phrases such as *clinical psychopharmacology* are attempts to solve the implied antagonisms. A breakdown of that term may help us to define our task: *Pharmacology* clearly pertains to the rational use of medicines in biological preparations and the study of their rates of absorption, excretion, sites of action, toxicity, etc. *Psycho* refers to the mind, *clinical* to ministrations at the bedside. Then, add to this the problems of development in childhood and we have a compound term that attests to the Anglo-Saxon origins of our English language. But, the reconciliation that really demands the most from us as physicians using medication is not linguistic; it concerns the fact that we not only have to bring together the mind, the body, and the behavior, but we also have to bring together these sectors in relation to a growing organism, in a changing social milieu with different requirements at different stages of the life cycle. The latter is what renders the developmental point of view unique from others and warrants a separate disciplinary definition, Child Psychiatry.

Development implies and includes concepts such as growth, differentiation, maturation, and, finally, integrated development itself. The first two terms are borrowed from biology, the third is a fiction of heuristic value to help us to make rational some of what we do. Growth pertains to the accretion of cells and changing size or mass; differentiation refers to specialization of more general cellular elements or differentiation of behavior from more global, syncretic beginnings to more highly specialized and articulated functions. Maturation refers to the natural unfolding of genetic potentials in "average expectable environments" (Hartmann, 1947). Development refers not only to maturation but also to the milieu in which maturation evolves. As such, development pertains to the species-specific potentials of an organism, and also to the variations in the environment at different stages and their resultants. The hierarchic structuralization of mind is the synthesis of all these forces impinging on an organism and serves as the background for creative and new behaviors in aging systems. In addition, child psychiatry includes affective components in its view of development, unlike some cognitive psychologies that exclude these factors to decrease the number of parameters to be considered in their experimental work.

While these general principles clarify some of the training biases of developmental psychiatrists, they do not cover the methodological biases that are inherent in the techniques used to study development. We can look at development from the standpoint of cross-sectional norms which indicate that this child ought to be this or that weight and height or have this and that variety of behavior at such and such an age. These normative approaches are characterized by varying testing devices which include I.Q., or D.Q., etc. Normalizing developmentalists of this ilk get bell-shaped distribution curves that show the relative presence or absence of behaviors in relation to chronological age. They are not usually interested in the structural underpinnings of changing capacity. There are also longitudinal techniques designed to alert us to the sequences and precursors of behavior in their increasing complexity as development ensues toward its ends as highly integrated and differentiated behaviors. In addition to these approaches, child psychiatrists also have been exposed to the concepts of ''developmental lines'' or ''aims of development'' outlined in terms of more general concepts of maturity not based on the *usual* but the *desirable* and *adaptive*. It is hard to separate such schemes from developmental Utopianism, but they are useful in pinpointing human capacity and its fulfillment. Anna Freud's scheme of developmental lines (1965) is one such program. Erikson (1963) offers another. He refers to the reconciliations that individuals are expected to make at each stage of development with their concomitant needs and capacities to adapt in an ecological balance with the rest of society and nature.

Our discussion to this point now presents us not only with the problem of bringing together substrate with behavior and epiphenomena of mind in consideration of the use of pharmacological agents, but also with various views of development which may not converge at the same focus. How can we reconcile these into a holistic program so that the child psychiatrist can still maintain the distinctiveness of his essential training as a developmental clinician? Clearly, such an approach would involve describing a process that is not so one-sided as to divide us into sectarian *organicists* or *functionalists* with their concomitant nasty definitions as ''brain changers'' or ''mind manipulators.'' Rather we should be able to describe a context in which we can function as physicians with a developmental bias that enables us to treat children as they are growing up with rational concern for their adaptation. In practice we see children with actual worries and wishes in real or imaginary trouble with a real environment of parents and society with similar or dissimilar desires and concerns. How can we succeed therapeutically using the enabling principles of our training?

DEVELOPMENTAL VIEW IN THEORY AND PRACTICE

A careful look at our peculiar training will enable us to outline further how we approach problems. We are all trained dualistically in medical schools as applied physiologists believing in the possibility of altering structure and function through mechanistic means, while at the same time we depend heavily on the doctor-patient relationship and the capacity of individuals to respond to talking, relationship, and insight therapies that range from psycho- to transactional analysis. It is exactly here that the developmental point of view does offer a conciliating felicity, because developmental principles not only tolerate the ambiguity of the presumed dualism, but offer theoretical reconciliations. Developmental observation does not permit a stand that is either all nature or all nurture. In order to make the variety of disorders we see in childhood understandable we have been trained to be alert to factors that we may (for sake of ease), call inner and outer influences. The weighting we give to each sector is highly dependent on the existing knowledge and information available within our science.

Freud's early interest in distinguishing *actual neuroses* from *psychoneuroses* revealed a strongly organismic and organic bias. On the other hand, the insistence on trauma as real and external showed his willingness to shift his focus to the external world as a source of pathological influence. Both of these concepts only came together when he explicated the notion of psychic reality and could postulate the possibilities of exploring the 'individual, who behaved neurotically.' Furthermore, when he made the etiological inferences about causes in the past, his guidelines for practice were posed as hypotheses yet to be tested.

Similarly we have seen an interesting history of changing concepts even within child psychiatry. A diagnosis such as "minimal brain dysfunction" is but one example of where we hedge our bets in reasoning by analogy to the presenting clinical picture of known organic mental syndromes with actual tissue damage. Yet, as child psychiatrists, we are aware that children bearing this formidable diagnosis can be helped clinically by a number of techniques which include substrate manipulation (medication) as well as learning techniques (tutoring) and frequently psychotherapy. Indeed, no one treatment is generally enough. When confronted by reality we are practical empiricists.

The adaptive point of view espoused by Hartmann and others talks about average biological equipment in an average expectable environment with a notion that the individual can come into homeostasis within himself as well as with his environment. He is fitted to adaptation in the ecological interplay within the family and the smaller community as well as the larger community if he is at least averagely endowed. *A thoroughgoing developmentalist must take the theoretical view that putting pressure on one sector in a system may gain effects within the same system but may also affect other systems.* Thus, a child psychiatrist must be alert to all sectors of development. When he uses drug therapy he is applying his skills to one sector alone but may affect the same or other sectors. In addition, the pharmacotherapy may not be sufficient by itself to affect all systems uniformly or beneficially.

In order to explicate these developmental principles, let us look at a number of practical examples commonly seen in child psychiatry and how the use of medication may alter the vital balance within and between subsystems and also require other therapeutic considerations.

During the second year of life, many children show interrupted sleep. The question frequently arises as to whether the child should be given some mild bedtime medication such as diphenhydramine (Benadryl). We have been told on the one hand that to do so might interfere with working out and arriving at a satisfactory resolution of a phase-specific conflict which may be operative in these infants. Their recent need to establish control, perhaps in response to toilet training or as a feature of the new negativism that emerges at the end of the second year, is clearly operative in some. While the drug may interfere with the mother-infant interface stimulated by a new training demand, the parents and the child are also in a balance developmentally. If the sleep disturbance interferes with the sense of well-being of the mother and her attitudes and concerns about the child, how will she respond to the continuing nighttime intrusions and will they evolve into a sense of battle? A sadomasochistic model could ensue from this eventuality as well as one where control is offered by a drug. "Would a mild sedative change the scenario to the developmental advantage of the infant at that level of patterning?" is the important question for a developmental psychopharmacologist.

At a still simpler level, we have been told that minimal brain dysfunction, especially in children who have encephalographic changes, is influenced favorably by the use of stimulant drugs (Satterfield et al., 1972; 1973). In fact, at this point in our knowledge, some argue that it may be reprehensible to hold back such medication in a child who needs help in focussing his attention in order to increase his learning potential. Not only do the matters that concern mother-child interface adhere as in the first instance, but we have also heard that there is a biological interface where the medication itself may have an effect on the growth potential of the child (Safer, 1973) and that interfering with one biological system must be considered in light of the benefits that the medication might offer. Again, each sector must be weighed within a full view of what is known about the other sectors.

In a more extreme circumstance such as childhood psychosis, the child who behaves bizarrely and has tantrums at times may be using his only adaptive means to bring himself to the attention of those who are his caretakers. We may be tempted to interfere with the radical behaviors, frequently at the behest of distraught parents. Should we do so if these are his only human interactions? At the interface of the child's interpersonal relations such an intervention (if it were possible to be handled with medication) would quiet the child, to be sure. However, we could not be certain that while the complaining environment might welcome the quieting, it might also deprive the child of the only attention he is, at that juncture, able to elicit. So often, medication is wrongly used to quiet, so as not to disturb, rather than as an adjunct to, or concomitant with, other methods designed to enhance developmental progress. These examples and others are presented only to bring to the attention of those who are interested in using medication for children that the medication alone is never sufficient. Parents and children's shorthand designations such as a ''reading pill'' are just as bad as the physician's ''he'll grow out of it,'' because each conveys the implication that one factor and one therapeutic intervention will suffice. The fact is that neither is salutary in itself without adjunctive help for other developmental systems participating in producing a well-functioning child in an adapted state with a minimum of useful anxiety.

The organismic view of development does not easily accede to dividing functions into varying sectors, but some more clarity may be gained by discussing each level of the human organization separately, largely on the justification that each level may be studied by a different method. This is done in light of a general caution that there is no mind without a brain, there is no behavior without stimuli, and childhood dependency is a feature of human development. These factors notwithstanding, we can look in a rational way at the individual child in relation to these varying sectors in order to explicate aspects of drug use according to known developmental principles.

We will first talk about biological development. We will then talk about developmental lines as the significant feature of the ego's adaptive organization and the influence of medication on such functions, and then take those functions which are more largely under the sway of the pleasure principle and look at the influence of drugs on fantasy formation, capacity for compromise, etc. Within each sector we will try to attend to the interactional homeostasis of the child at each stage of development with reference to his caretakers, ranging from mother through teacher and reaching to the extended community. Their developmental expectations and normative values will be looked at as feeding back to and influencing the maturing and developing child. The overall developmental view of the changing meaning of a developing child to his parents and community as well as the changing meaning of varying techniques available for modulating development will be examined with special reference to the use of medication.

INDEPENDENT AND INTEGRATED SECTORS OF DEVELOPMENT

1. Biological Features

The child is in a biological process of growth, maturation, and development. These may be measured by any of the techniques of anthropometrics such as height and weight curves, physiological responses that clinically include blood pressure and pulse rate, temperature control, etc., or at the biochemical level by the techniques that are available for observing the changes that occur in liver and thyroid function with progressive chronological maturation. In addition, whatever single function is potentially affected by any medication can itself be monitored along with behavior. In order to keep close track on developmental biological issues, one must have a working knowledge and empirical understanding of the supposed sites of action of each drug as well as their potential side effects, and utilize available measures as a means of monitoring both drug dosage and drug effectiveness. Because we are interested in behavioral alterations, it is all too easy to forget that the medication itself works on a biochemical substrate and that the substrate alteration may be sufficiently distressing to warrant changing either the drug used or its dosage.

A developmentally alert clinician will also attend to the biological sectors that require influence because slow psychological development may be secondary to slow physical maturation. When looking for target symptoms to influence by drugs, the clinician must consider the organism's developmental underpinnings. For example, poor socialization in early adolescence may accrue in part from late development of secondary sexual characteristics (McCandless, 1960).

Another important developmental factor to be considered is that although we may be altering an undesirable developmental trait by medicating, there may be secondary effects of the drug which are less desirable. For example, fluorides are useful to strengthen the enamel of teeth, but they also may lead to mottling which is unsightly later in life. Chlorpromazine is certainly useful as an antipsychotic neuropleptic but also has a tendency to lower the seizure threshhold; it is often sedating at therapeutic dosage levels and may interfere with learning.

The third factor to be considered among biological factors concerns the natural thrust of maturation itself which is relatively independent of external environmental influences. Methodologically we must always ask whether it is the medication we have given the child that is providing the change or do we have development and maturation on our side to do the job? Is it the specificity of the particular agent or the general attention-focussing effect it provides? A child, for example, who has not gained a function, such as speech, who begins to speak while the drug is being administered can provide us with the "therapeutic fallacy" that "the drug did it." Our certainty has to be tempered with developmental skepticism and then the progressive encouragement of more careful ways of controlled measurement of results. Moreover, when a developmental landmark is achieved during the pharmacologic treatment of the child, it not only could be argued that the medication did it, or set it in motion, but it may be that the child had attained a critical hierarchic integration and can now go ahead on his own steam without further need for a boost. These are the factors which lead us to question whether or not medications ought to be discontinued intermittently; to question whether or not their long-term effects are or are not desirable; and whether interruption will negate the new ground gained. Our models must include "developmental boosters" designed to prod development along, "developmental sustainers" designed to modulate development on a continuous basis, and placebos which function as "environmental suggestives" to permit auxiliary support to children in human milieus.

Even a biological view of development depends on behavioral scaling for evidence of effectiveness. As physicians, we know it is not enough to treat the diabetic's urine but the patient with diabetes. We may look at children as having a number of characteristics from infancy on that require monitoring. Many investigators have chosen their own favorites (Fries, 1953; Fish, 1967; Thomas and Chess, 1963). I would choose four as having particular biological significance: Anergy-energy, modulated-unmodulated, attention-inattention, and predictive patterning versus randomness. From the developmental point of view, each of these features may be a factor in temperamental and characterological disposition. One expects that as development proceeds there will be an increasing balance among all these sectors: The child ought to be energetic enough, sufficiently modulated and attending in his behavior, and with predictable rhythmicity. We expect that he may have periods of crankiness and difficulty and show decreases in attention at times, but with the increasing demands of society as he develops, the general trend should be toward more predictability in balance and toleration of frustration as well as capacity for pleasure.

When using medication one has to have in mind some norms in these sectors but also be prepared to allow leeway for stylistic variation. For example, the attention span of an infant of six months is clearly shorter than the attention span of a two-year-old who may be operating within the context of the omnipotence of the practicing period as described by Mahler et al. (1975). Yet such a child's attention disposition may be quite short and he may be apparently unresponsive to societal demands as compared to the attention span available to a four-year-old who is expected to attend and even cooperate in a nursery program. Clinicians would have to take into account the richness of variation in children's behavior that may be based on maturational biological factors but also on other influences, when they consider whether or not a medication should or ought to be used. One would not want to convert *exuberance* to *hyperactivity* by *interpretation of the meaning* of behaviors, because exuberance would be desirable whereas hyperactivity is definitionally fraught with undesirable connotations.

2. Behavioral Measures

Now we must again confront the difficulty alluded to before of assaying which method or model of development we should use as a yardstick to measure drug effect on behavior? There are many global severity rating scales available; there are also checklists of symptoms available; there is the developmental lines vantage point. One can even break development into hypothetical stages such as libidinal organization or ego integrations. Any or all of these methods have and may be used to verify change, but we ought to recognize that changes that take place at one level of development might not be considered desirable or may even be undesirable at another, and also that any checklist or global scale omits features present in others. For example, many checklists have an item for "separating easily from the parent." This is desirable at three and a half or four if nursery school is the order of the day, but one would like to see protest and separation anxiety in a nine- to thirteen-month-old as an index of attachment behavior, which we consider a significant prognosticator of future object relations. Similarly, just because in our current state of culture we send our children to school at three or four, enlightened teachers do not expect our children to be able to play reciprocally at age three. Moreover, the measure of a developmental landmark thus must be seen in the context of the demands of the teacher coordinated with the requirements of the home. "Sesame Street" and similar environmentally enriched cognitive nutriments may invite, even excite the child to read at three, but we certainly would agree with Piaget and others that it is not necessary that he begin to read at three, so long as he achieves the age-appropriate developmental landmarks for cognitive development when "their time comes." Moreover, early reading does not guarantee enjoyment from reading. Indeed, Piaget has often quipped that the American question is "can we do it earlier," whereas he is more interested in the invariance of and processes underlying the sequences of development which enable reading and other skills. While we are able to pick up reading disabilities earlier and earlier, there are currently no decent predictive studies that would suggest that we are so accurate in who or which child will have a frank reading disability from those who do well, even with their minimal perceptual lags. From a developmental standpoint, the issue is one of distinguishing a lag in maturation from a fixed or developmental "lesion."

3. Nonnormative Developmental Lines Approach

Generally, child psychiatrists utilize a broader definition of developmental disorders than the simple normative index of the presence of symptoms, or cognitive deficits. Some functions are clearly in the biological maturational scheme of things but these interact with other psychic and social structures too. A truly developmental position within psychiatry looks at symptom formation that is not of this developmental variety as way-stations in solving conflicts not only with the external world, but also within. There may be transient identifications or transient compromises that result in new ego adaptations. Enuresis provides an interesting example of a common symptom that may have a number of roots and may be examined developmentally. Some families insist that the child be placed on the potty as soon as he can sit and use "gastrocolic reflexology" as their ally in toilet training, figuring that bladder training follows bowel training. Other families, on the advice of enlightened physicians, insist that the 'myelinization route' be followed and that one should not put pressure on a child until it reaches eighteen months when the sphincter is supposedly innervated. Other families who feel children should never be coerced do not really toilet train their children and trust that somehow the socialization process will include toilet training by shame or social constraint. With this environmental variability of possible impositions, or lack of impositions, on the child the central notion of the move from body tyranny to body control as a developmental line has gained in attractiveness to developmentally alert clinicians. When is the child able to participate in the control of his bowels and bladder for his own purposes becomes the central query for such a frame of reference.

In yet another vein, at what stage and in what kind of community should we expect the child to have less separation anxiety rather than more, and in what communities would it be wiser if the child stuck close to an adult's side because of the actual dangers in his environment? To what degree should a child be expected to yield his egocentric wishes and move toward more cooperative approaches when it is possible that one or the other of the approaches is valued in his particular community? However, maturation also may make a child more capable of moving away from his own primary demands towards social demands. If we accept Piaget's frame of reference, it is a distinct step in development when the child can decentrate and take the other individual's vantage point cognitively. Does this, itself, influence the capacity to move out of the egocentric position or is it a prerequisite to achieving the social step of cooperation?

This brief excursion into the developmentalists' language now permits a better framework for understanding drug use in children.

If parents and/or schools ask for drugs as an adjunct in helping the over-assertive, egocentric, unsocialized child they may in fact be asking for a drug to increase the speed of development of a cognitive process that may be slower in this specific child on a maturational basis. It may be that the use of the drug for nonpharmacological effects in quieting the complaining community or school may influence the child indirectly by a trickle-down effect resulting in a less threatened and anxious child. Clearly, the facts are that ego developmental lines or ego functions themselves will be only secondarily influenced by medication, insofar as medications somehow affect the substrate, the background music, the noise factor, the resultant anxiety that underlies the symptoms that may accrue. On the other hand, a relieved community puts less pressure on a child.

The developmental line of movement from body to toy to work enables us to observe a gradual reorganization of a child's thinking as well as the encroachment of reality factors on pleasure factors. These can be directly inferred clinically from the vantage point of "capacity to attend to play," which might be considered an ego function, and also from inferences concerning how much and what kind of libidinal or aggressive organizations are expressed in the fantasies themselves. This could lead us to a method of understanding the drive factors from the standpoint of how a drug modulates wishes and what the balance is in a regression-progression continuum. Moreover, such observation can be used to interpret how the child distortedly or realistically interprets the medication itself and how it fits into his fantasies.

First we may inquire on a cognitive level whether the child is using predominantly mediational or associational thinking, and whether his level is appropriate and normal for his stage of development. Second, we may assay the "relative abundance" of aggressive themes. Third, is there too much fusion or diffusion of drives. Moreover, we can observe how much expression of the drive is tolerated as opposed to dampened and inhibited, and how this expression emerges relative to expectations at each developmental stage. As clinicians, we have certain normative standards of how well a child ought to be able to control or express his fantasies. All in all, we are looking for the happy balance at each stage and age that represents an appropriate equilibrium between drive factors and their organization in goal-oriented wishes as these accrue in an adaptive relationship in accord with the requirements of the community in which the child lives.

For some children the pressures of wishes may be insistent, persistent, and oppressive to their own sense of well-being. For other children the inhibitions may be strong, because of excessive social demands. Either of these states (too much or too little) may lead the clinician to prescribe medication. Usually, in neurotic compromises there is a tendency to dampen excessively and create substitutive symptoms which in themselves reveal a pressure similar to the drives, as in obsessional questioning or tics. However, when drives in the form of bizarre fantasies encroach on reality, a child may act in an uninhibited manner that tends to disrupt his relationships to peers and adults alike. Clinicians should be neither activity makers nor dampeners but seek to establish better homeostatic mechanisms from within that ultimately can be trusted. The developmental notion that modulation from without has to be replaced by controls from within is another form of this developmental proposition. We assume that as ego apparatuses develop, gratification of the drives become possible in and along socially acceptable channels and that each stage of development is seen to have its appropriate pleasures and controls.

4. The Meaning of Taking Drugs

If a child's fantasies are laden with aggression and fears of penetration and/or oral impregnation, the administration of a medication taken by mouth may be fraught with unhappy meaning for that child. According to his capacity for reality testing, he may fancy that he is being poisoned, that one is putting foreign substances into him, that he is being given a magical strengthening potion, etc. If the mother is in charge of the drug administration, she may be looked upon as the object from whom the evil or balm is dispensed. Giving medication also may be perceived according to prior patterns of interaction in families; for example, as a continuation of an earlier pattern of oral assault—being forced to eat, or being duped into a dishonest relationship. The background of basic trust would have to be assessed before one entrusts a mother to participate in medicating a child and before one decides that it is she rather than the child himself who is to administer it. If the level of conflict is centered about toilet training, giving drugs can deteriorate into a sadomasochistic struggle, or taking medicine can be construed as pleasing mother by being submissive. Contrariwise, administration of drugs may become a nonparticipating pseudoalliance enveloped in denial of passivity.

Other means of giving medication as by injection or suppository form offer even more possibility for misinterpretation. Anal sadistic assault is easily read into such routes. Phallic level interpretations may be dominant no matter what the route of administration. The notion of being intruded on, seduced, or having one's manhood taken away or femininity mocked are all possible modes of interpretation for a vulnerable child who has been made to feel less than adequate by whatever symptom he has that requires pharmacological treatment.

The hope that fantasy life and reality organization will become modulated by the administration of medication also depends on what life problems have to be solved by the child at what stage of his development.

SUMMARY

A drug used to treat a symptom without some understanding of the nature of the disorder in developmental terms is not only poor clinical practice, but also antithetical to the developmental propositions that guide the work of child psychiatrists. These developmental principles mesh with the old pharmacological rule of thumb that suggests one use the appropriate drug in the appropriate dose for the right child who has a given symptom that is the target for a desired effect. Developmentally, we must add the caution that the drug be used for as long a time as necessary and titrated to the current needs of our patients based on what is known to be different about them because they are children.

Not only must a child be considered at each stage of his development for his maturity in accepting the medication but also for the maturity of his detoxification methods—his routes of absorption and excretion and end-organ responses. The therapeutic effects expected must be potentially better than the toxic or side effects and the therapeutic toxic ratio must be satisfactory for the stage of development of the young patient. One cannot simply compare the responses of adults to the responses of children. We must take into account the 'paradoxical' differences that accrue at different stages of development and which may be very discreetly demarcated by chronological (maturational) age (Fish, 1967). Extrapolation of dose by body weight simply does not apply in children, just as indices of severity are more important than diagnosis per se. Level of I.Q. will also be determining because as psychic organization becomes more complex, drug effect is less clearly dependent on biological effect. For example, Diphenhydramine is well tolerated in very high doses with good effect on modulating behavior until age ten, following which it may have the same soporific effect as on adults and more importantly not effect the target behavior. Moreover, it tends to be effective in the disorders of minor severity. Developmentally, we are required to look at toxicity not only as toxicity to the physiological biological system but toxicity in the sense of behavioral deterioration which interferes with the desired "good functioning" of the child (Fish and Shapiro, 1964). Again, this diversion into biology amidst a discussion of psychological factors points up the need to look for developmental balance, not simple effects on one sector of behavior. Parents must be guided not only by their wish that the child lose a symptom, but by the fact that the symptom may signify developmental turmoil or temperamental variety as well as an indicator of pathology.

One must also be guided by the fact that the use of medication is something that is neither desirable or undesirable in itself according to preconceived notions, but something that may help to achieve an aim in helping a child grow up to be able to accept the opportunity that is available educationally and socially. If a clinician can bring a parent into this kind of cooperative participation, drug therapy will be infinitely more successful and less prone to possible failure due to conflict between the child and his parents or parents and physician. While a physician may have authority on his side and want to provide placebo effect by lending the weight of that authority, he must always take into consideration that overselling a medication leads to disappointments for the parents as well as the children and encourages a lack of confidence for future therapeutic enterprises.

The developmentally alert clinician should maximize his therapeutic relationship before any medication is used. This requires careful and prolonged consultation as well as accurate dose-regulation in a particular child. Now, because there are an increasing number of pharmacological agents being touted as effective for troubled behavior, children will be subjected to an increasing likelihood of having drugs offered to take care of their problems by practitioners, many of whom are not psychiatrically sophisticated. If the public mind associates giving drugs to children with the illegal and illicit "drug scene" a detrimental effect is projected onto the possibility for influencing the therapy of children who need medication and who may otherwise be subjected to prolonged suffering. Moreover, if a contaminated view of drug administration prevails within the family, the developmental effect on the growing child will be to establish attitudes against a "pill pushing" culture. On the other hand, careless and promiscuous drug administration will lead to disillusionment, cynicism, and gross neglect for many children who are medicated and not otherwise treated. Attention to the process of drug administration in the context of developmental principles as outlined should make the administration of medication for children more reasonable and provide a framework of limits, aims, and constraints as well as a well-tempered appropriate optimism.

References

Erikson, E. H. (1963), *Childhood and society,* 2nd Ed. New York: Norton, pp. 247–274.

Fish, B., and Shapiro, T. (1964), A descriptive typology of children's psychiatric disorders: II. A behavioral classification in child psychiatry. *APA Psychiat. Res. Rep., 18;* 75–86.

Fish, B. (1967), Methodology in child psychopharmacology. In D. H. Efron et al. (Eds.), *Psychopharmacology, review of progress.* Public Health Publ. No. 1836.

Freud, A. (1965), *The concept of developmental lines. Normality and pathology in childhood: Assessments of development.* New York: Int. Univ. Press, pp. 56–92.

Fries, M., and Woolf, P. (1953), Some hypotheses on the role of congenital activity type in personality development. *Psychoanalytic Study of the Child.* New York: Int. Univ. Press, *8,* 48–62.

Hartmann, H., Kris, E., and Loewenstein, R. M. (1947), Comments on the formation of psychic structure. *Psa. Study of the Child.* New York: Int. Univ. Press, pp. 11–38.

McCandless, B. (1960), Rate of development: Body build and personality. In *Child development and child psychiatry. APA Psychiat. Res. Rep.,* No. 13, p. 42.

Mahler, M. (1952), On child psychosis and schizophrenia: Autistic and symbiotic infantile psychoses. *Psa. Study of the Child.* New York: Int. Univ. Press, pp. 286–305.

Mahler, M. S., Pine, F., and Bergman, A. (1975), *The psychological birth of the human infant.* New York: Basic Books.

Safer, D. J., and Allen, R. P. (1973), Factors influencing the suppressant effects of two stimulant drugs on the growth of hyperactive children. *Pediatrics, 51,* 660–667.

Satterfield, M. D., Cantwell, D. P., and Lesser, L. I. (1972), Physiological studies of the hyperkinetic child. I *Am. J. Psychiat., 128;* 1418–1424.

Satterfield, H. H., Lesser, L. I., and Saul, R. E. (1973), EEG aspects in the diagnosis and treatment of minimal brain dysfunction. *Ann. N.Y. Acad. of Sci., 205,* 274–282.

Thomas, A., Chess, S., Birch, H. G., Hertzig, M. E., and Korn, S. (1963), *Behavioral individuality in early childhood.* N.Y. Univ. Press.

Part II

THE CLINICAL
APPLICATIONS

Chapter Five

TREATMENT OF CHILDHOOD AND ADOLESCENT SCHIZOPHRENIA [1]

Magda Campbell, M.D.

INTRODUCTION

The efficacy and superiority of neuroleptics over psychosocial treatments alone in schizophrenia of adults has been confirmed (GAP, 1975; Klein and Davis, 1969). These drugs not only diminish individual symptoms, but also affect the course of the illness (WHO, 1967).

Relatively good agreement on diagnostic criteria for adults and the use of large numbers of subjects in collaborative studies has greatly contributed to the availability of a vast body of knowledge (for review, see Klein and Davis, 1969). Acquisition of such information has been possible because treatments were compared in samples of patients as homogeneous as possible concerning diagnosis, duration of illness, and other pertinent variables. With sophisticated methodology it has been possible to separate the responders to a drug from the nonresponders, even within a major diagnostic category such as depressive illness.

Such is not the case in psychotic children and adolescents who are designated schizophrenic. Numerous factors have contributed to the unsatisfactory state of psychopharmacology in this age group. Only the following factors will be discussed here: methodology in clinical drug trials, prognosis of illness, size of samples, diagnosis and classification.

Methodology of Psychopharmacology

With the exception of research conducted in the hyperkinetic MBD child, studies in the young age group of psychiatric patients often are poorly controlled and lack appropriate rating instruments sensitive enough to reflect changes. Methodology in childhood psychopharmacology has been reviewed elsewhere (Campbell, 1975a, forthcoming; Conners, 1973; Eisenberg, 1964; Fish, 1968, 1969; *Psychopharmacology Bulletin,* 1973; Sprague and Werry, 1971), and methodological considerations are discussed in greater detail in ch. three.

The outcome of drug treatment is influenced by the natural history of illness— its severity and duration, the child's chronological age, maturation, development, I.Q., and parental influences (Fish, 1968).

The first step in the assessment of therapeutic efficacy of drugs is usually a *single dose study.* The next stage of investigation is frequently an *open study,* if the safety and efficacy of a single dose has been established to the investigator's satisfaction. If the drug shows therapeutic effectiveness, a more formal *clinical trial* is conducted. The methodology of clinical drug trials, including considerations of randomization, matching, single-subject design, crossover design and double-blind conditions, is discussed by Conners in ch. three. For the assessment of baseline behavior and for the measurement of change due to drug administration, psychiatric rating scales, standardized, sensitive, and appropriate for the patient population are required (for review, see Campbell, in press, and Conners, ch. three).

Before starting the drug, an adequate period (two to three weeks) of placebo administration is necessary to ensure the excretion ("washout") of prior medication. This will also get both patient and nurse into the routine. The same procedure can be used in an attempt to identify placebo responders before the administration of an "active drug" (Jones and Ainslie, 1966). Adequate length of placebo interval is also required between two drug conditions in crossover studies.

Rating conditions are crucial for critical assessment of drug efficacy, particularly in younger age groups. The use of independent multiple raters, who observe the patient under different conditions (classroom, home, or hospital ward) is strongly recommended.

The method of determining the appropriate dosage is a controversial issue. The Bellevue group, based on experience with psychotic children, recommends individual dose regulation, starting with low, often ineffective doses. Escalation should be gradual, at regular intervals (once or twice a week) until positive or untoward effects are observed, and only then is the optimal dose determined.

General principles of clinical trials and methods of establishing statistical significance are further reviewed and discussed by Bradford-Hill (1971).

Prognosis of Illness

No currently available drug or any other treatment for that matter, will result in dramatic improvement or changes in a severely impaired young autistic child, or a school-age child or adolescent who has continuously shown severely deviant development and behavior since earliest life (Bender, 1967; Eisenberg, 1956; Kanner, 1971; Rutter, 1970; Quitkin, Rifkin, and Klein, 1976). The guarded prognosis limits the efficacy of the currently available drugs in these subgroups of psychotic patients.

Samples

The subjects in drugs studies which have been published are often not only behaviorally poorly defined, but samples are often heterogeneous with regard to diagnosis and age. Schizophrenics are considered together with the mentally retarded who have some behavioral problems. Furthermore, the samples are invariably small. All this has made it difficult, if not impossible, to draw valid conclusions regarding the therapeutic efficacy of psychotropic agents in the treatment of childhood schizophrenia. Research, particlarly involving new drugs, is usually conducted with inpatients. Unfortunately, most psychiatric divisions in large medical centers affiliated with universities lack inpatient units for children.

Diagnosis

This remains an unresolved problem, although efforts have been made to spell out diagnostic criteria (for review, see Goldfarb, 1970; Rutter, 1967; Wing, 1966). In 1933 Potter outlined six diagnostic criteria for schizophrenic children, two of which are clearly derived from symptoms manifested by adults (dereistic thinking and disturbances of thought) and are not applicable to young, retarded psychotics. Bradley and Bowen (1941) used more descriptive, and therefore objective criteria. These included both primary or necessary (seclusiveness and irritability) and secondary symptoms, eight altogether. Bender (1947, 1956) offered more a theoretical frame of reference, though of inestimable value, than an empirical list of symptoms. Kanner (1943) described infantile autism, a psychosis of early childhood (starting before the second birthday), characterized by disturbance of affective contact, failure to use speech for communication, and maintenance of sameness, among other symptoms. The British working party (Creak, 1964) outlined nine diagnostic points, chiefly derived from Kanner (1943), but encompassing all forms of childhood psychosis. These points are: withdrawal from people; apparent unawareness of own personal identity to a degree inappropriate to age; preoccupation with certain objects; resistance to change; abnormal perceptual experience; seemingly illogical anxiety—while appropriate sense of fear in the face of real danger may be lacking; speech never acquired or lost, echolalia, mannerisms of use and diction; various abnormalities of motility, including hyper- or hypokinesis and bizarre stereotypes; and the last, a background of retardation in which islets of normal, near normal, or exceptional intellectual function or skill may appear.

Rutter (1966, 1967) objected to two of the nine points, finding anxiety and hyperactivity to be nonspecific, and gave a more detailed listing of behavioral characteristics for early childhood psychosis.

In children, or adolescents, with a relatively normal development prior to manifestation of schizophrenia, the symptoms resemble those seen in adults: they are chiefly the Bleulerian basic symptoms, disturbance of affect and thought. However, as far as the accessory symptoms are concerned, the prepuberty child will have introjects and the voices are only later projected and experienced as hallucinations.

In this author's experience, the behavioral manifestations will depend on the maturational-organizational level of the individual; this has been stated by others (Fish and Shapiro, 1965; Wolff and Chess, 1964).

Classification and Its Relationship to Drug Response

In this chapter the term psychosis will be used for schizophrenia and/or infantile psychosis (or autism) only. These disorders are known in DSM II (1968) as schizophrenia, including schizophrenia, childhood type; and in GAP (1960) as early infantile autism, interactional psychotic disorder (psychoses of infancy and early childhood), schizophreniform psychotic disorder (psychoses of later childhood), and schizophrenic disorder, adult type (under psychoses of adolescence).

These psychotic disorders of childhood and adolescence can be divided into three broad groups on the basis of age of onset (Eisenberg, 1967; Rutter, 1967). The first group consists of patients in whom the psychotic disorder is manifested in infancy or occasionally as late as the second or even the third year of life (Eisenberg, and Kanner, 1956; Kanner and Lesser, 1958). The second type of psychosis usually begins at the age of three to five, after relatively normal development to that time. Patients belonging to a third type show manifestations of psychosis shortly before puberty or in early adolescence.

This is not an etiological classification, but it may be useful in terms of phenomenology, course of illness, and prognosis.

It is beyond the scope of this chapter to discuss the pros and cons of this classification. Several authors in the field (Eisenberg, 1972; Kolvin, 1971; Rutter, 1972) maintain that these are independent disease entities. Others (Bender, 1967, 1975; Fish, 1971) have not made these distinctions. Fish (1971) proposed that "the clinical picture can be related to the time of life when development is disrupted. A different pattern of assets and handicaps is produced, depending on which function was emerging or due to emerge, at the time development became disorganized. . . . The severity of the lags and disorganization in development also varies. In general, when the early transient neurological disturbances are the most severe, there is greater interference with later intellectual and social adaptive functioning and less capacity for defense formation. The most severe early impairments are less modifiable by the pharmacologic or nonpharmacologic treatment'' (477–78).

Thus, the earlier the onset of illness, the more globally the individual child may be affected, and this will be manifested not only by disturbed behavior but often also may be associated with mental retardation and central nervous system dysfunction.

In a comparative study of early and late onset of childhood psychoses, Kolvin (1971) showed that the infantile psychotic group (early onset) had significantly higher occurrence of perinatal complications, neurologic and electroencephalographic abnormalities, and seizures than the late onset group. In other words, the evidence of cumulative cerebral damage or dysfunction was markedly greater in children who showed evidence of severe developmental disorder since earliest life. Others too have found a preponderance of organicity in the early onset psychosis (Rutter and Lockyer, 1967), and abnormal neurologic findings in early infancy were found to be precursors of psychological aberrations in the later life of schizophrenics (Fish, 1957, 1975).

Goldfarb divided schizophrenic children into two subgroups on the basis of their pre- and perinatal history and neurologic findings (1961, 1974).

It is possible to delineate two distinct subgroups within adolescent and young adult schizophrenics on the basis of premorbid history, academic and social competence, I.Q., and neurologic status (Quitkin, Rifkin, and Klein, 1976). The two groups show differential response to drug treatment (Klein, 1967, 1968). Such differential drug response was also found in small samples of preschool age psychotic children (Campbell et al., 1972a; Campbell et al., 1976; Fish et al., 1968). These are initial observations, and need replication and amplification in studies with patients carefully selected and well defined. On the other hand, various indicators of neurologic dysfunction were found more frequently in schizophrenic children and adolescents than in nonschizophrenics or normal children (Birch and Hertzig, 1967; Gittelman and Birch, 1967; Hertzig and Birch, 1966, 1968).

There is some indication that a psychoactive drug capable of producing behavioral improvement in schizophrenics, including adolescents, may also alter positively biochemical and psychological parameters (Brambilla and Penati, 1971; Brambilla et al., 1974).

For adolescents who show the clinical picture of acute schizophrenia, the purpose of treatment is to restore normal functioning. For the two- to four-year-old child, with onset of psychosis in infancy, one would like not only to restore functioning to normal, but also promote the delayed or retarded development. Emerging or nonexistent functions, such as speech and adaptive skills, have to be created. Whereas in adults and adolescents with acute schizophrenia, diminution in reactivity via neuroleptics is desirable (Himwich, 1960), the same is considered an untoward effect in the young child who is apathetic, anergic, and lacking any motor initiative.

On the basis of her clinical experience and research, Fish (1970) found that the prepuberty psychotic child is comparable to the chronic schizophrenic adult in terms of response to drugs. Thus, the child may be sedated by small doses of the sedative type of neuroleptics, and the more stimulating agents will evoke a more therapeutic response.

On the other hand, a small portion of very young and low I.Q. children respond positively to psychoactive agents that cause worsening of psychosis in the adult schizophrenic (Campbell, Fish, Shapiro, and Floyd, 1971a; Campbell, Fish, Korein, Shapiro, Collins, and Koh, 1972b; Campbell, Small, Collins, Friedman, David, and Genieser, 1976). Thus, there is some, though not yet conclusive, evidence that psychoactive agents may be related to the pathophysiology of psychosis in children and adolescents:

1. The more severely disturbed and impaired (low I.Q.) patients require potent psychoactive agents such as the neuroleptics; they respond less favorably or even fail to respond to treatment with milder drugs, such as diphenhydramine (Fish, 1960; Fish and Shapiro, 1964, 1965). Less impaired psychotic children may show clinical improvement even on placebo (Fish and Shapiro, 1964, 1965) or milieu treatment (Fish, Shapiro, and Campbell, 1966). Fish suggested that in high I.Q. schizophrenics, diphenhydramine be tried as a first step in drug treatment because of its safety and the ease with which it can be regulated.

2. Clinical experience has shown that the prepuberty, particularly the preschool-age psychotic child, is often excessively sedated by the aliphatic type of phenothiazines (chlorpromazine) on doses which diminish some of the symptoms (Campbell, Fish, Korein, Shapiro, Collins, and Koh, 1972b; Campbell, Fish, Shapiro, and Floyd, 1972c; Fish, 1960, 1970). The piperazine type of phenothiazine (trifluoperazine) with its stimulating actions, proved to be somewhat better in that respect (Fish et al., 1966). The youngest age group of schizophrenic patients respond to drugs in similar fashion as the adult chronic schizophrenics who are anergic, apathetic, and withdrawn (Fish, 1970). These findings led to a series of drug trials, including psychoactive agents with stimulating properties, which were safe and effective in the adult counterpart of these children (Campbell, Fish, Shapiro, and Floyd, 1970, 1971a, b, 1972; Campbell, Fish, Korein, Shapiro, Collins, and Koh, 1972b; Campbell, Fish, David, Shapiro, Collins, and Koh, 1972a, 1973; Campbell, Small, Collins, Friedman, David, and Genieser, 1976; Fish, Campbell, Shapiro, and Floyd, 1969a).

It is conceivable that the excessive sedation of the child at very low doses of chlorpromazine, for example, may be a result of the degree of cerebral dysfunction.

3. Some children with early onset of psychosis respond with clinical improve-

ment to psychoactive agents which usually cause worsening of symptoms in adult schizophrenia, particularly in acute types. This too may be related to differences in pathophysiology, if not etiology (Campbell, Fish, Shapiro, and Floyd, 1971; Campbell, Fish, Korein, Shapiro, Collins, and Koh, 1972b; Campbell, Small, Collins, Friedman, David, and Genieser, 1976).

INDICATIONS

There is no evidence which is based on well-controlled studies that drug treatment is more effective in schizophrenic children and adolescents than any other type of treatment, nor has it been demonstrated that drug administration is more effective when combined with some other treatment modality (for review, see Campbell, in press). However, experience has shown that drug treatment can be a valuable addition or an essential modality in the total treatment of the schizophrenic child, particularly in the adolescent with acute onset of psychosis.

Neuroleptics are most effective in diminishing psychomotor excitement. This is a direct effect on a target function of behavior and usually predictable. The indirect effect develops slowly, probably as a result of the modified interaction of the individual with the environment (Irwin, 1968). The only enduring effects of drug therapy on behavior are due to these concurrent environmental psychosocial treatments. The hyperactive child with short attention span, when calmed down by a drug, may be able to focus his attention on a task and thus acquire some reading and writing skills. The agitated, assaultive, or self-mutilating patient, when these symptoms are eliminated or reduced with an effective psychoactive medication, may develop more adaptive social interactions that, in turn, will improve learning. Drugs themselves do not create learning or intelligence, nor do they necessarily alter parental attitude, but they can make the patient more amenable to environmental treatments or manipulations. It is important to institute drug treatment in the early stage of illness rather than after other, frequently inappropriate, therapies have failed. Though this was not systematically investigated, in our clinical experience, patients seemed to respond more to drug therapy in the early stages of illness.

Clearly, in the formative years of the individual, drugs alone never suffice. The choice of other treatments (environmental manipulations, remedial education, individual psychotherapy, group therapy, parental counseling), as well as hospitalization, will depend on contributing factors, associated handicaps of the individual patient, and the family. Many patients, even after the cessation of symptoms such as hyperkinesis, agitation, hallucinations—and no longer in need of drug therapy—will require continuation of other treatment(s) and follow-up.

CLASSIFICATION AND DOSAGE OF NEUROLEPTICS

Phenothiazines

The phenothiazines are divided into three subclasses: aliphatic, piperidine, and the piperazine derivatives. The aliphatic group (chlorpromazine, triflupromazine) produce sedative-hypnotic effects. This may be desirable in an older child or an adolescent with acute psychosis and associated symptoms of agitation and assaultiveness. Such diminution of reactivity is not therapeutic in the young apathetic and anergic child, where psychosis is often associated with retarded functioning. The purpose of treatment in this group of patients is not only to normalize disorganized functions, but skills such as speech and other adaptive behaviors which are absent, have to be created. In these cases, a more stimulating piperazine derivative, such as trifluoperazine or fluphenazine, is recommended. Thioridazine is the representative of the piperidine subclass. It has a low incidence of extrapyramidal and autonomic side effects, and seems to be well tolerated by individuals with preexisting seizure disorders (Freeman, 1970).

Chlorpromazine can be given orally in two to four divided doses, from 9 to 200 mg./day in children under twelve years of age. Doses in adolescents are comparable to adult doses. The maximum dose intramuscularly up to five years of age is 40 mg. The dose range of *thioridazine* is comparable to that of chlorpromazine. The total daily dosage of triflupromazine ranges from 1 to 150 mg.

Fluphenazine and *trifluoperazine* (FDA approval for patients over six years of age only) can be given in doses of 0.25 mg. up to 16 mg. daily, in one to two doses.

Thioxanthenes [2]

Chlorprothixene (FDA approval for patients over six years of age only) can be given in a single dose, or divided, from 10 to 200 mg. daily. *Thiothixene* (FDA approval for patients over twelve years of age only) is given in one to two doses a day, from 1 to 40 mg. daily. This class of drugs is less likely to produce hematopoetic and hepatic damage and photosensitivity reactions than the phenothiazines. Thiothixene has stimulating properties and a wide therapeutic margin.

Butyrophenones [3]

This class of drugs decreases agitation without the hypnotic effect of aliphatic phenothiazines. However, the incidence of extrapyramidal side effects is high.

Haloperidol (FDA approval for patients over twelve years of age only) has been found effective in both withdrawn and assaultive or self-mutilating patients. It can be given in a single dose or in divided doses, from ½ mg. to 16 mg. daily.

Dihydroindolones [4]

Data indicate that *molindone* (FDA approval for patients over twelve years of age only) is a neuroleptic with some characteristics of antidepressants (activating and stimulating properties, like the piperazine phenothiazines). With the exception of extrapyramidal side effects, it causes fewer untoward reactions than aliphatic and piperidine phenothiazines. To the present time, only one report on its efficacy in children has been published (Campbell, Fish, Shapiro, and Floyd, 1971b; for review, see Ayd, 1975a).

DRUG ADMINISTRATION AND SPECIAL CONSIDERATIONS
IN THE YOUNG

Fish (1967) pleaded that before instituting drug therapy, the relation of the patient and his symptoms to his family be assessed. The patient's response to outpatient or institutional psychiatric treatment should be evaluated for two to four weeks before beginning medication. Such a baseline period of observation is not feasible in emergency situations.

A careful inquiry into drug allergy or sensitivity, as well as a comprehensive history of prior drug intake (type of drug, dosage, duration, and date of last drug administration) must be obtained. This is of utmost importance, particularly in emergency situations, since drug potentiation may take place. Therefore, for an emergency, chloral hydrate or paraldehyde (oral or intramuscular) should be used rather than a neuroleptic.

The choice of drug will depend on many factors. Barbiturates and diphenylhydantoin should not be used in the treatment of psychoses. They are ineffective and may cause a worsening of disorganization.

Diphenhydramine, in divided doses, starting with 30 mg./day up to 800 mg./day, may be used as the first drug. If the patient does not respond, a neuroleptic should be tried.

Although many neuroleptics are in use today, it is sufficient to be familiar with one or two from each class or subclass. As a rule, the most familiar and seasoned drug should be tried first, that is, a *phenothiazine*. *Chlorpromazine* or *thioridazine* is effective, particularly in cases of marked hyperactivity or agitation. When symptoms such as apathy and anergy predominate, a stimulating type of neuroleptic such as *trifluoperazine* is indicated. Although the superiority of one class of neuroleptics over another in the treatment of schizophrenia has not been demonstrated, an individual patient may respond more favorably to another class of neuroleptics than to a phenothiazine. However, before switching to another drug, it should be determined whether the lack of therapeutic response is due to failure of the parent to administer the drug or failure of the patient to ingest the medication.

A patient refractory to a phenothiazine or responding to small doses with excessive sedation should be given a trial of *thiothixene, haloperidol,* or, last, *molindone,* in that order.

The latest edition of the PDR should be consulted concerning drug administration to children under twelve years of age.

The parents, and the patients, with the exception of very young or retarded children, should be informed as to expected therapeutic effects, possible adverse effects of the drug, and dose regulation, as well as to the limitations of drug treatment. The availability of the treating physician, even by telephone, may prevent serious complications as well as unnecessary anxieties. If the parents are uncooperative or unreliable, neuroleptics or other potentially harmful drugs should not be prescribed on an outpatient basis. Accidental overdosage in young children and impulsive suicidal gestures in adolescents with medically prescribed drugs occur frequently.

Great individual differences among children have been found so far as optimal dose is concerned. The dosage is frequently unrelated not only to age and weight, but even to severity of symptoms or illness (Fish, 1968). Doses in adolescents are comparable to adult doses. Medication should be started with a low dose, usually therapeutically ineffective. Increments should be gradual, weekly, until the symptoms decrease, disappear, or untoward effects are noted, and then the optimal dose determined. Within the limits of compliance with the most recent PDR, full dose exploration for each patient is essential because of the individual differences, some of which might be due to differences in absorption or metabolism. Underdosage involves most of the risks of medication without the therapeutic benefits. Nevertheless, it is poor medicine to maintain the patient on excessively high doses of drugs that interfere with functioning and may result in long-term complications.

Of the *untoward effects,* particularly in children, the first to be seen frequently are the behavioral. Some of the undesired effects (sleepiness or hypoactivity) are exaggerated forms of desired effects. Overdosage may result in worsening of preexisting symptoms (hyperactivity, irritability), and must be differentiated from too low a dose.

The *immediate* untoward effects of neuroleptics, in addition to behavioral toxicity (alteration of psychomotor and perceptual-cognitive functions and emotional states—for review, see Di Mascio and Shader, 1970; Di Mascio, Shader, and Giller, 1970) are cutaneous disorders, hepatic damage, agranulocytosis and extrapyramidal effects. These latter include parkinsonian reactions (mask-like faces, drooling, cogwheel phenomenon, and tremor), acute dystonic reactions (dystonias, dyskinesias, oculogyric crisis, myoclonic twitchings, protrusion of tongue, opisthonos, torticollis, and dysarthria), and akathesia (inability to be still). For a detailed review, see Greenblatt, Shader, and Di Mascio (1970).

Untoward effects due to excess drug can be eliminated by decreasing the dosage. At times the medication may have to be discontinued for a day or two. Untoward effects may occur on the optimal dose due to drug accumulation or because lowering of dosage may be required consequent to clinical improvement.

Parkinsonian side effects are seen less frequently in young children than in adolescents. Lowering the dosage is suggested rather than the routine administration of antiparkinsonian agents; there is evidence that these drugs decrease the plasma levels of neuroleptics and their clinical efficacy (for review see Ayd, 1975b). For the relief of acute dystonic reactions administration of 25 to 50 mg. of diphenhydramine intramuscularly or orally is effective. Hepatic and hematopoetic damage is infrequent in this young age group under careful clinical and laboratory monitoring.[5]

Phenothiazines generally lower seizure threshhold. There is evidence that chlorpromazine increases seizures in patients with a prior history of convulsive disorder (Tarjan, Lowery, and Wright, 1957). Induction of seizures seems to be less frequent by the piperidine phenothiazines; thioridazine actually seems to be beneficial in the treatment of behavioral disorders of children with convulsive disorders (Freeman, 1970; for review, see Di Mascio, Soltys, and Shader, 1970). Anticonvulsants can be administered, if necessary, in conjunction with the neuroleptic.

Information concerning *long-term untoward effects* is limited. Since psychoactive agents affect the neurotransmitters which control the secretion of hypothalamic neurohormones, caution should be exercised in their administration to prepubertal children and adolescents. They may influence growth, central nervous, endocrine, and reproductive systems. Chlorpromazine decreases growth hormone secretion in adults (Sherman, Kim, Benjamin, and Kolodny, 1971); there are no reports on children. Menstrual irregularities, amenorrhea, galactorrhea, aspermia, and particularly marked weight gain have been noted. Prolonged administration of neuroleptics may affect I.Q. (McAndrew, Case, and Treffert, 1972).

Reports are available concerning a neurologic syndrome in children resembling tardive dyskinesia in adults (Moline, 1975; Schiele, Gallant, Simpson, Gardner, and Cole, 1973). McAndrew, Case, and Treffert (1972) found that of 125 hospitalized patients, aged eight to fifteen years, ten developed involuntary movements of the upper extremities with akathesia *after* the abrupt withdrawal of phenothiazines. In addition, six patients showed facial tics. These neurological effects were first observed three to ten days after drug withdrawal. They ceased within three to six months. Comparison of these ten patients with those who remained asymptomatic showed that the median duration of drug intake was thirty-two months in the symptomatic group, versus four months in the asymptomatic group. The daily termination dose was 400 mg. of chlorpromazine equivalents, in accordance with the standard dose conversion table (Hollister, 1970) in the symptomatic and only 99 mg. in the asymptomatic group. The median gram intake was 403 in the first and 8.7 grams in the latter group.

Polizos, Engelhardt, Hoffman, and Waizer (1973) found that fourteen out of thirty-four outpatient childhood schizophrenics showed similar symptoms (involuntary movements, primarily in the extremities, trunk and head, associated with ataxia) after withdrawal of neuroleptics, which included haloperidol and thiothixene. Both abrupt total withdrawal and gradual, graded withdrawal with weekly reduction of dose by 25 percent gave the same results. The relationship of this apparently reversible syndrome to persistent, tardive dyskinesia in adults has not been determined (Engelhardt, 1974).

Ocular (lenticular, corneal, and retinal) symptoms are rarely seen in children.

For a detailed review of drug side effects, a chapter by Shader (1970), a book by Shader and Di Mascio (1970), and the latest edition of the PDR are recommended.

Failure of drug response can be due to a variety of factors which include noncompliance, underdosage, overdosage, polypharmacy, drug absorption, metabolism, or genetic determinants (for review, see Ayd, 1975b). If a drug fails to induce a therapeutic response after four to eight weeks of administration, another drug from the same or another class of neuroleptics should be tried, as suggested earlier.

The physician's limited knowledge of psychopharmacology is a frequent cause of "drug treatment resistance" in patients, depriving them of an effective and relatively economic treatment modality. However, one must keep in mind that there are individual patients whose symptoms are refractory to drug treatment.

Duration of drug treatment has to be judged on an individual basis. Drug administration should not be continued unless necessary. Four to six weeks of drug maintenance may suffice for acute psychoses. Each three to four months, after gradual lowering of dosage, the drug should be discontinued for a week or two, and the patient's clinical status reassessed. Medication should be reinstituted if symptoms recur. Shorter drug-free periods or "drug holidays" are recommended over weekends, or when feasible, as during school vacations. It is believed that intermittent discontinuation of neuroleptics will reduce both the risks and incidence of adverse reactions. Clinical experience has shown that drug-induced positive behaviors and developmental gains can be retained even after drug withdrawal.

Neuroleptics should be discontinued during acute febrile or common childhood illnesses. After the patient has fully recovered, medication should be reinstituted in gradual increments.

RESEARCH NEEDED

Psychopharmacology of schizophrenic children and adolescents is still in a primitive state. The literature has been reviewed by Campbell (1973, 1975a, b), Werry (1972), and Freeman (1970). Drug studies with large samples of homogeneous populations, controlled for age, I.Q., and other pertinent variables, are needed. Such studies can be carried out only in collaborative trials.

The populations should be defined, not only by behavioral diagnostic criteria, but also by other parameters. These include demographic profile, family history of schizophrenia, pre- and perinatal insult to central nervous system, electroencephalogram, clinical evidence of central nervous system dysfunction (including performance I.Q.), and biochemical profile.

Drug response should be evaluated in subgroups with acute and insidious onset, with and without evidence of central nervous system dysfunction.

Drug effects should be assessed not only on behavior, but also on other parameters, such as electroencephalogram, biochemistry, and performance tasks. The purpose of such investigations is to determine why some patients respond to a drug and others do not. It is essential to delineate possible responders from nonresponders.

Drug studies should be designed to distinguish direct drug effect on target functions (arousal, motor activity, and others) from indirect effects which result from interaction with the environment (Turner, Purchatzke, Gift, Fanner, and Uhlenhuth, 1973).

The immediate and long-term effect of drugs on cognitive functions should be critically assessed. Long-term efficacy studies on behavior are essential to understand the proper role of drugs in treatment. Long-term monitoring of drugs may disclose their untoward effects on various systems, including the endocrine and central nervous system.

Stimulating psychoactive agents should be investigated in subgroups or individuals who fail to respond to the standard neuroleptics.

The efficacy of drug treatment should be compared to placebo and to psychosocial therapies (psychotherapy, milieu therapy, behavior therapy, etc.), and drug therapy should be explored in conjunction with psychosocial therapies.

Above all, anterospective studies of the natural history of psychoses with and without pharmacologic intervention are needed.

CONCLUDING REMARKS

There has been little systematic investigation of the role of chemotherapy in the treatment of childhood and adolescent schizophrenia. For this, the unsatisfactory state of diagnosis, classification, and methodology can be faulted, among other factors.

Currently available therapeutically effective drugs are not viewed as a long-term treatment modality, but rather as a temporary, though often essential, adjunct. Hopefully the drug will make the growing and developing patient more amenable to other treatments which comprise the total treatment.

The possible hazards of chemotherapy have to be weighed against the hazards of untreated illness, or ineffectiveness of some lengthy, usually costly, and often unavailable therapies.

There is some supportive evidence that clinical distinctions may be correlated or even improved by certain demographic, biochemical, neurophysiologic, and endocrine criteria to determine which subtypes of the mixed population of young psychotics may benefit from a drug. Until this is achieved, chemotherapy remains on an empirical basis.

Correlations of behavior manifestations with these parameters may not only imply important genetic and other biological abnormalities in these populations and define drug responders from nonresponders, but such an approach may result in better understanding of the disease itself.

Notes

1. Part of this work was supported by Public Service Grant MH-04665 from the National Institute of Mental Health. The author is grateful to Richard I. Shader for helpful comments.
2. Suggested reading: Campbell, Fish, Korein, Shapiro, Collins, and Koh, 1972; Engelhardt, Polizos, Waizer, and Hoffman, 1973; Faretra, Dooher, and Dowling, 1970; Fish, 1960, 1970; Fish, Campbell, Shapiro, and Floyd, 1969b; Fish and Shapiro, 1964, 1965; Fish, Shapiro, and Campbell, 1966; Korein, Fish, Shapiro, Gerner, and Levidow, 1971.

3. Suggested reading: Campbell, Fish, Shapiro, and Floyd, 1970; Simeon, Saletu, Saletu, Itil, and Da Silva, 1973; Waizer, Polizos, Hoffman, Engelhardt, and Margolis, 1972; Wolpert, Hagamen, and Merlis, 1967.

4. Suggested reading: Engelhardt, Polizos, Waizer, and Hoffman 1973; Faretra, Dooher, and Dowling, 1970, Lewis and James, 1973; Pool, Bloom, Mielke, Roniger, & Gallant, 1976.

5. Pretreatment alkaline phosphatase, serum glutamic-pyruvic transaminase (SGPT), serum glutamic-oxaloacetic transaminase (SGOT), complete blood count (CBC), and urinalysis are recommended. These tests are to be repeated weekly during the first two months of treatment, once a month until the sixth month, and thereafter when indicated.

References

Ayd, F. J. (1975a), Moban: The first of a new class of neuroleptics. In F. J. Ayd (Ed.), *Rational psychopharmacotherapy and the right to treatment*. Baltimore: Ayd Medical Communications, Ltd., pp. 91–105.

Ayd, F. J. (1975b), Treatment resistant patients: A moral, legal and therapeutic challenge. In F. J. Ayd (Ed.), *Rational psychopharmacotherapy and the right to treatment*. Baltimore: Ayd Medical Communications Ltd., pp. 37–61.

Bender, L. (1947), Childhood schizophrenia: Clinical study of 100 schizophrenic children. *Am. J. Orthopsychiat.*, *17*, 40.

Bender, L. (1956), Childhood schizophrenia: 2. Schizophrenia in childhood—its recognition, description and treatment. *Am. J. Orthopsychiat.*, *26*, 499–506.

Bender, L. (1967), Theory and treatment of childhood schizophrenia. *Acta Paedopsychiat. 34*, 298.

Bender, L. (1975), A career of clinical research in child psychiatry. In E. J. Anthony (Ed.), *Explorations in child psychiatry*. New York: Plenum Press, pp. 419–462.

Birch, H. G., and Hertzig, M. E. (1967), Etiology of schizophrenia: An overview of the relation of development to atypical behavior. In: *The origins of schizophrenia*. Proceedings of the First Rochester International Conference 29–31 March, 1967. *Excerpta Medica International Congress*, Series No. 151, pp. 92–110.

Bradford-Hill, A. (1971), *Principles of medical statistics*. New York: Oxford Univ. Press.

Bradley, C., and Bowen, M. (1941), Behavior characteristics of schizophrenic children. *Psychiatric quarterly, 15,* 298–315.

Brambilla, F., Guerrini, A., Riggi, F., and Ricciardi, F. (1974), Psychoendocrine investigation in schizophrenia. *Dis. Nerv. Sys., 35,* 362–367.

Brambilla, F., and Penati, G. (1971), Hormones and behavior in schizophrenia. In D. H. Ford (Ed.), *Influence of hormones on the nervous system*. Basel: Karger, pp. 482–492.

Campbell, M. (1973), Biological interventions in psychoses of childhood. *J. Aut. & Ch. Schiz., 3,* 347–373.

Campbell, M. (1975a), Pharmacotherapy in early infantile autism. *Biol. Psychiat., 10,* 399.

Campbell, M. (1975b), Psychopharmacology in childhood psychosis. In R. Gittelman-Klein (Guest Ed.), Recent advances in child psychopharmacology. *Int. J. Ment. Health, 4,* 238–254.

Campbell, M. (forthcoming), Psychopharmacology for children and adolescents. In J. D. Noshpitz (Ed.), *Basic handbook of child psychiatry*. New York: Basic Books.

Campbell, M., Fish, B., David, R., Shapiro, T., Collins, P., and Koh, C. (1972a), Response to triiodothyronine and dextroamphetamine: A study of pre-school schizophrenic children. *J. Aut. & Ch. Schiz., 2,* 343.

Campbell, M., Fish, B., Korein, J., Shapiro, T., Collins, P., & Koh, C. (1972b), Lithium and chlorpromazine: A controlled crossover study in hyperactive severely disturbed young children. *J. Aut. & Ch. Schiz., 2,* 234.

Campbell, M., Fish, B., David, R., Shapiro, T., Collins, P. & Koh, C. (1973), Liothyronine treatment in psychotic and non-psychotic children under 6 years. *Arch. Gen. Psychiat., 29,* 602.

Campbell, M., Fish, B., Shapiro, T., and Floyd, A. (1970), Thiothixene in young disturbed children, A pilot study. *Arch. Gen. Psychiat., 23,* 70.

Campbell, M., Fish, B., Shapiro, T., and Floyd, A. (1971a), Imipramine in preschool autistic and schizophrenic children. *J. of Aut. & Ch. Schiz., 1,* 267.

Campbell, M., Fish, B., Shapiro, T., and Floyd, A. (1971b), Study of molindone in disturbed preschool children. *Curr. Ther. Res., 13,* 28.

Campbell, M., Fish, B., Shapiro, T., and Floyd, A. (1972c), Acute responses of schizophrenic children to a sedative and "stimulating" neuroleptic: A pharmacologic yardstick. *Curr. Ther. Res., 14,* 759.

Campbell, M., Small, A. M., Collins, P. J., Friedman, E., David, R., and Genieser, N., (1976), Levodopa and levoamphetamine: A crossover study in schizophrenic children. *Curr. Ther. Res., 19,* 70–86.

Chassan, J. B. (1960), Statistical inference and the single case in clinical design. *Psychiat., J. for the Study of Interpersonal Processes, 23,* 173.

Conners, C. K. (1973), Deanol and behavior disorders in children: A critical review of the literature and recommended future studies for determining efficacy. *Psychopharmacology Bulletin.* Special Issue, Pharmacotherapy of children. NIMH, 1973, p. 188. DHEW Publication No. (HSM) 73-9002.

Creak, M. (1964), Schizophrenic syndrome in childhood: Further progress report of a working party. *Dev. Med. and Ch. Neurol., 4,* 530–535.

Diagnostic and statistical manual of mental disorders, 2nd Ed. (DSM-II), APA, 1968.

Di Mascio, A., and Shader, R. I. (1970), Behavioral toxicity, Part I. Definition and Part II. Psychomotor functions. In R. I. Shader, and A. Di Mascio (Eds.), *Psychotropic drug side effects.* Baltimore: Williams and Wilkins Co., pp. 124–131.

Di Mascio, A., Shader, R. I., and Giller, D. R. (1970), Behavioral toxicity, Part III. Perceptual-cognitive functions and Part IV. Emotional (mood) states. In R. I. Shader, and A. Di Mascio (Eds.), *Psychotropic drug side effects.* Baltimore: Williams and Wilkins Co., pp. 132–141.

Di Mascio, A., Soltys, J. J., and Shader, R. I. (1970), Psychotropic drug side effects in children. In R. I. Shader, and A. Di Mascio (Eds.), *Psychotropic drug side effects,* Baltimore: Williams and Wilkins, pp. 235–260.

Eisenberg, L. (1956), The autistic child in adolescence. *Am. J. of Psychiat., 112,* 607.

Eisenberg, L. (1964), Role of drugs in treating disturbed children. *Children, 2,* 167.

Eisenberg, L. (1967), Psychotic disorders in childhood. In L. P. Eron (Ed.), *The classification of behavior disorders.* Chicago: Aldine.

Eisenberg, L. (1972), The classification of childhood psychosis reconsidered. *J. of Aut. & Ch. Schiz., 2,* 338–342.

Eisenberg, L. and Kanner, L. (1956), Early infantile autism, 1943–55. *Am. J. of Orthopsychiat., 26,* 556–566.

Engelhardt, D. M. (1974), CNS Consequences of psychotropic drug withdrawal in autistic children: A follow-up report. Presented at the Annual ECDEU Meeting, Key Biscayne, Florida, May 23–25.

Engelhardt, D. M., Polizos, P., Waizer, J., and Hoffman, S. P. (1973), A double-blind comparison of fluphenazine and haloperidol in outpatient schizophrenic children. *J. of Aut. & Ch. Schiz., 3,* 128.

Faretra, G., Dooher, L., and Dowling, J. (1970), Comparison of haloperidol and fluphenazine in disturbed children. *Am. J. of Psychiat., 126,* 1670.

Fish, B. (1957), The detection of schizophrenia in infancy. *J. of Nerv. and Ment. Dis., 125,* 1–24.

Fish, B. (1960), Drug therapy in child psychiatry: Pharmacological aspects. *Comp. Psychiat., 1,* 212.

Fish, B. (1967), Organic therapies. In A. M. Freedman and H. I. Kaplan (Eds.), *Comprehensive textbook of psychiatry.* Baltimore: Williams and Wilkins Co., p. 1468.

Fish, B. (1968), Methodology in child psychopharmacology. In D. H. Efron, J. O. Cole, J. Levine, and J. R. Wittenborn (Eds.), *Psychopharmacology, review of progress, 1956–1967.* Public Health Service Publication No. 1836, p. 989.

Fish, B. (1970), Psychopharmacologic response of chronic schizophrenic adults as predictors of responses in young schizophrenic children. *Psychopharm. Bull., 6,* 12.

Fish, B. (1971), Contributions of developmental research to a theory of schizophrenia. In J. Hellmuth (Ed.), *Exceptional infant,* Vol. 2. *Studies in abnormalities.* New York: Brunner/Mazel Inc., pp. 473–482.

Fish, B. (1975), Biological antecedents of psychosis in children. In D. X. Freedman (Ed.), *The biology of the major psychoses: A comparative analysis.* Ass. Res. Nerv. Ment. Dis. Publ. No. 54. New York: Raven Press.

Fish, B., and Shapiro, T. (1964), A descriptive typology of children's psychiatric disorders, II. A behavioral classification. *APA Psychiat. Res. Rep., 18,* 75.

Fish, B., and Shapiro, T. (1965), A typology of children's psychiatric disorders, I. Its application to a controlled evaluation of treatment. *J. Am. Acad. Ch. Psychiat., 4,* 32.

Fish, B., Shapiro, T., and Campbell, M. (1966), Long-term prognosis and the response of schizophrenic children to drug therapy: A controlled study of trifluoperazine. *Am. J. Psychiat., 123,* 32.

Fish, B., Shapiro, T., and Campbell, M. (1968), A classification of schizophrenic children under five years. *Am. J. Psychiat., 124,* 1415.

Fish, B., Campbell, M., Shapiro, T., and Floyd, A. (1969a), Schizophrenic children treated with methysergide (Sansert), *Dis. Nerv. Sys., 30,* 534.

Fish, B., Campbell, M., Shapiro, T., and Floyd, A. (1969b) Comparison of trifluperidol, trifluoperazine and chlorpromazine in preschool schizophrenic children: The value of less sedative antipsychotic agents. *Curr. Ther. Res., 11,* 589.

Freeman, R. D. (1970), Psychopharmacology and the retarded child. In F. Menolascino (Ed.), *Psychiatric approaches to mental retardation.* New York: Basic Books, p. 294–368.

Gittelman, M., and Birch, H. G. (1967), Childhood schizophrenia. *Arch. Gen. Psychiat., 17,* 16–25.

Goldfarb, W. (1961), *Childhood schizophrenia.* Cambridge: Harvard Univ. Press.

Goldfarb, W. (1970), Childhood psychosis. In P. H. Mussen (Ed.), *Carmichael's manual of child psychology,* 3rd Ed., Volume II. New York: John Wiley and Sons, pp. 765–830.

Goldfarb, W. (1974), *Growth and change of schizophrenic children: A longitudinal study.* New York: Halsted Press Book, John Wiley and Sons.

Greenblatt, D. J., Shader, R. I., and Di Mascio, A. (1970), Extrapyramidal effects. In R. I. Shader, and A. Di Mascio (Eds.), *Psychotropic drug side effects.* Baltimore: Williams and Wilkins Company, pp. 92–106.

Group for the Advancement of Psychiatry (GAP) (1966), *Psychopathological disorders in childhood: Theoretical considerations and a proposed classification,* Vol. VI, Report No. 62.

Group for the Advancement of Psychiatry (GAP) (1975), *Pharmacotherapy and psychotherapy: Paradoxes, problems and progress,* Vol. IX, Report No. 93.

Hertzig, M. E., and Birch, H. G. (1966), Neurologic organization in psychiatrically disturbed adolescents. *Arch. Gen. Psychiat., 15,* 590–598.

Hertzig, M. E., and Birch, H. G. (1968), Neurologic organization in psychiatrically disturbed adolescents. *Arch. Gen. Psychiat., 19,* 528–537.

Himwich, H. E., Kety, S. S., and Smythies, J. R. (1967), *Amines and schizophrenia.* New York: Pergamon Press.

Hollister, L. E. (1970), Choice of antipsychotic drugs. *Am. J. Psychiat., 127,* 186.

Irwin, S. (1968), A rational framework for the development, evaluation, and use of psychoactive drugs. *Am. J. Psychiat., Supp., 124,* 1.

Jones, M. B., and Ainslie, J. D. (1966), Value of placebo wash-out. *Dis. Nerv. Sys., 27,* 393.

Kanner, L. (1943), Autistic disturbances of affective contact. *Nervous Child, 2,* 217–250.

Kanner, L. (1971), Follow-up study of eleven autistic children originally reported in 1943. *J. Aut. & Ch. Schiz.,* 1, 119.

Kanner, L., and Lesser, L. I. (1958), Early infantile autism. *Ped. Clin. of N. Am., 5,* 711–730.

Klein, D. F. (1967), Importance of psychiatric diagnosis in prediction of clinical drug effects. *Arch. Gen. Psychiat., 16,* 118–126.

Klein, D. F. (1968), Psychiatric diagnosis and a typology of clinical drug effects. *Psychopharmacologia, 13,* 359–386.

Klein, D. F., and Davis, J. M. (1969), *Diagnosis and drug treatment of psychiatric disorders.* Baltimore: Williams and Wilkins Co.

Kolvin, I. (1971), Psychoses in childhood—A comparative study. In M. Rutter (Ed.), *Infantile autism: Concepts, characteristics, and treatment.* Edinburgh: Churchill Livingstone, pp. 7–26.

Korein, J., Fish, B., Shapiro, T., Gerner, E. W., and Levidow, L., (1971), EEG and behavioral effects of drug therapy in children: Chlorpromazine and diphenhydramine. *Arch. Gen. Psychiat., 24,* 552.

Lewis, P. J. E., and James, N. Mcl. (1973), Haloperidol and chlorpromazine: A double-blind crossover trial and clinical study in children and adolescents. *Australian and New Zealand J. of Psychiat., 7,* 59.

McAndrew, J. B., Case, Q., and Treffert, D. (1972), Effects of prolonged phenothiazine intake on psychotic and other hospitalized children. *J. Aut. and Ch. Schiz.*, *2*, 75.

Moline, R. A. (1975), Atypical tardive dyskinesia. *Am. J. Psychiat.*, *132*, 534–535.

Polizos, P., Engelhardt, D. M., Hoffman, S. P., and Waizer, J. (1973), Neurological consequences of psychotropic drug withdrawal in schizophrenic children. *J. Aut. & Ch. Schiz.*, *3*, 247.

Pool, D., Bloom, W., Mielke, D. H., Roniger, J. J., and Gallant, D. M. A controlled evaluation of loxitane in seventy-five adolescent schizophrenic patients. *Curr. Ther. Res.*, *19*, 99–104.

Potter, H. W. (1933), Schizophrenia in children. *Am. J. Psychiat.*, *12*, 1253–1270.

Psychopharmacology Bulletin (1973), Special Issue, Pharmacotherapy of children. NIMH. DHEW Publication No. (HSM) 73-9002.

Rutter, M. (1966), Behavioural and cognitive characteristics of a series of psychotic children. In J. K. Wing (Ed.), *Early childhood autism*. Oxford: Pergamon Press, pp. 51–81.

Rutter, M. (1967), Psychotic disorders in early childhood. In A. J. Coppen, and A. Walk (Eds.), *Recent developments in schizophrenia: A symposium*. London: R.M.P.H., pp. 133–158.

Rutter, M. (1970), Autistic children: Infancy to adulthood. *Seminars in Psychiat.*, *2*, 435–450.

Rutter, M. (1972), Childhood schizophrenia reconsidered. *J. Aut. & Ch. Schiz.*, *2*, 315–337.

Rutter, M., and Lockyer, L. (1967), A five to fifteen year follow-up study of infantile psychosis. I. Description of sample. *Brit. J. of Psychiat.*, *113*, 1169–1182.

Quitkin, F., Rifkin, A., and Klein, D. (1976), *Neurologic soft signs in schizophrenia and character disorders. Arch. Gen. Psychiat.*, *33*, 845–853.

Schiele, B. C., Gallant, D., Simpson, G., Gardner E., and Cole, J. O. (1973), Tardive dyskinesia. *Am. J. Orthopsychiat.*, *43*, 506.

Shader, R. I. (1970), Endocrine, metabolic, and genitourinary effects of psychotropic drugs. In A. Di Mascio, and R. I. Shader (Eds.), *Clinical handbook of psychopharmacology*. New York: Science House, pp. 205–212.

Shader, R. I., and Di Mascio, A. (Eds.) (1970), *Psychotropic drug side effects*. Baltimore: Williams and Wilkins Co.

Sherman, L., Kim, S., Benjamin, F., and Kolodny, H. (1971), Effect of chlorpromazine on serum growth-hormone in man. *New Eng. J. Med.*, *284*, 72.

Simeon, J., Saletu, B., Saletu, M., Itil, T. M., and DaSilva, J. (1973), Thiothixene in childhood psychoses. Presented at the Third International Symposium on Phenothiazines, Rockville, Maryland.

Sprague, R. L., and Werry, J. S. (1971), Methodology of psychopharmacological studies with the retarded. In N. R. Ellis (Ed.), *International review of research in mental retardation*. New York: Academic Press, 148.

Tarjan, C., Lowery, V. E., and Wright, S. W. (1957), Use of chlorpromazine in two hundred seventy-eight mentally deficient patients. *AMA J. Dis. Ch.*, *94*, 294.

Turner, D. A., Purchatzke, G., Gift, T., et al. (1973), Intensive design in evaluating anxiolytic agents. Presented at a Symposium on Clinical Pharmacological Methods, New Orleans, La.

Waizer, J., Polizos, P., Hoffman, S. P., Engelhardt, D. M., and Margolis, R. A. (1972), A single-blind evaluation of thiothixene with outpatient schizophrenic children. *J. Aut. & Ch. Schiz.*, *2*, 378.

Werry, J. S. (1972), Childhood psychosis. In H. C. Quay, and J. S. Werry (Eds.), *Psychopathological disorders of childhood*. New York: John Wiley and Sons, pp. 173.

Wing, J. K. (1966), Diagnosis, epidemiology, aetiology. In J. K. Wing (Ed.), *Early childhood autism*. Oxford: Pergamon Press, pp. 3–49.

Wolff, S., and Chess, S. (1964), A behavioral study of schizophrenic children. *Acta Psychiat. Scand.*, *40*, 438–466.

Wolpert, A., Hagamen, M. B., and Merlis, S. (1967), A comparative study of thiothixene and trifluoperazine in childhood schizophrenia. *Curr. Ther. Res.*, *9*, 482.

World Health Organization (WHO) (1967), *Scientific group on psychopharmacology: Research in psychopharmacology*. Tech. Rep. Series No. 371. Geneva: World Health Organization.

Chapter Six

PSYCHOPHARMACOLOGIC TREATMENT OF THE MINIMAL BRAIN DYSFUNCTION SYNDROME

Dennis P. Cantwell, M.D.

INTRODUCTION

This chapter will discuss the psychopharmacologic treatment of children with the syndrome of minimal brain dysfunction. However, before this central topic of the chapter can be examined, several problem areas must be reviewed. These include: terminology, classification, and definition of the syndrome; the diagnostic evaluation of these children; and general problems in evaluating drug treatment of childhood disorders.

TERMINOLOGY AND CLASSIFICATION

Terms such as "brain-damage syndrome" (Strauss and Lehtinen, 1947), "minimal brain damage" (Gesell and Amatruda, 1949), "minimal brain dysfunction" (Clements, 1966), "hyperkinetic syndrome" (Cantwell, in press), and "hyperactive child syndrome" (Stewart et al., 1966) are often used synonymously. Since these terms have been used in widely divergent ways by different investigators, the same children have been described by different terms and different children by the same terms. Thus, research findings cannot be readily compared. Moreover, the terms "brain-damage syndrome," "minimal brain damage," and "minimal brain dysfunction" imply etiology, while terms such as the "hyper-kinetic syndrome" and "hyperactive child syndrome" are behavioral descriptions.

If "brain damage" is used in its literal sense to mean structural abnormality of the brain, the "brain-damage syndrome" is an inaccurate and misleading term for the condition under discussion. While some children who present with the clinical picture of hyperactivity or hyperkinesis may suffer from demonstrable brain damage, it is clear that the majority do not (Werry, 1972). Likewise, most brain-damaged children do not present with the clinical picture of the hyperki-netic syndrome, although they are at risk for the development of psychiatric problems (Rutter et al., 1970a).

"Brain dysfunction" may be a more accurate term than "brain damage" to describe those children who present with less well-defined disorders manifested by more subtle neurological signs. These more subtle alterations in coordination, perception, or language may only occasionally be associated with actual damage to the brain (Rutter, 1968). Moreover, many hyperkinetic children do not dem-onstrate even these subtle neurologic signs. Thus "brain dysfunction syndrome" may be an inappropriate term to describe the large percentage of hyperactive children who present primarily with behavioral abnormalities. Finally, techniques for the reliable and accurate quantification of "brain dysfunction" in children are not available. Yet prefixing the word "minimal" to "brain dysfunction" implies just such a quantification.

Perhaps the most comprehensive and clearest exposition of the term "minimal brain dysfunction" is put forth by Wender (1971). Wender postulated five clini-cal subgroups of the "minimal brain dysfunction syndrome":

1. Hyperactive child
2. Neurotic child
3. Psychopathic child
4. Schizophrenic child
5. Child with specific learning disabilities

Wender justified grouping together these five categories of children with het-erogenous clinical pictures by postulating the same "core" underlying pathophy-siology. He speculated that there may be a biochemical basis to this underlying pathophysiology (Wender, 1975).

In contrast, the hyperactive child syndrome (or hyperkinetic syndrome) is a behavioral syndrome with specified behavioral criteria for diagnosis. The author has suggested elsewhere (Cantwell, 1975b) that the core symptoms of this syn-drome are: hyperactivity, distractibility, and short attention span, impulsivity, and excitability. Additional symptoms commonly seen in many, but not all, hyperactive children include: antisocial behavior, specific learning disabilities, and emotional symptoms such as depression and low self-esteem. While it is simpler to diagnose this condition than to diagnose the much more heterogenous condition of "minimal brain dysfunction," it should be pointed out that difficulties exist in definition and measurement of such items as "hyperactivity" and "short attention span" (Klein and Gittelman-Klein, 1975).

Two separate organizations are presently considering the problem of the definition and classification of this syndrome. The World Health Organization seminars on classification in child psychiatry has proposed a multi-axial classification scheme (Rutter et al., 1969; Tarjan and Eisenberg, 1972). Recently Rutter and his colleagues recommended a multi-axial scheme with five axes (Rutter et al., 1974): 1. the clinical psychiatric syndrome; 2. the child's current level of intellectual functioning, regardless of etiology; 3. specific developmental disorders; 4. associated or etiological biological factors; 5. any associated or etiological psychosocial factors. This five-axis scheme is also being considered for the American Psychiatric Association Diagnostic and Statistical Manual, 3rd Ed. (DSM-III). The Rutter group recommended retaining the term "hyperkinetic syndrome of childhood." The DSM-III group, however, feeling that the short attention span and the distractibility are the essential features of the syndrome, has recommended that the term "attentional deficit disorder" replace the terms "hyperkinetic syndrome" and "minimal brain dysfunction." Subcategories recommended by the DSM-III group are:

1. uncomplicated
2. with hyperactivity
3. with conduct problems
4. with conduct problems and hyperactivity

The majority of children with this syndrome would have specific developmental disorders, particularly reading retardation, listed on axis three of the multi-axial classification. However this clinical syndrome is also known to be common in children with low I.Q. (Pond, 1961), with frank brain damage (Ingram, 1956), and with epilepsy (Ounsted, 1955). These factors would be classified in the appropriate way on axes two and four. Clinical studies of the parents of children with the hyperkinetic syndrome indicate that a significant percentage were themselves hyperkinetic as children and are psychiatrically disturbed as adults (Morrison and Stewart, 1971; Cantwell, 1972). In these cases the appropriate notation would be made on axis five. Unanswered as yet is whether the syndrome occurring in children with a low I.Q., or with evidence of frank brain damage, or with psychiatrically disturbed parents is a different condition than the syndrome occurring in children with no evidence of abnormalities on two, three, four, and five. Present evidence suggests that the term "minimal brain dysfunction" is used to describe a heterogeneous group of children with different clinical pictures and probably different etiologies for their condition. The clinical disorder may be due to a structural abnormality of the brain (Werry, 1972), or an abnormality of physiological arousal of the nervous system (Satterfield et al., 1974); in others there may be a genetic basis for the disorder (Cantwell, 1975a); while in others there may be still-undiscovered important etiologic factors. An elucidation of specific etiologic factors for different groups of children presenting clinically with this syndrome is a task for future research and will allow subclassification of the syndrome based on etiology.

In this chapter, this more restricted concept of the minimal brain dysfunction syndrome describing the hyperactive or hyperkinetic child will be used. While Wender's conception of the five clinical subtypes with the same underlying pathophysiology may be correct, hard evidence for this view is lacking at present. Moreover most of the drug studies of children with "minimal brain dysfunction" have been conducted on children fitting the more narrow description.

EPIDEMIOLOGY AND NATURAL HISTORY

Epidemiologic studies indicate that the syndrome may occur in as many as 5 to 10 percent of prepubertal children with the boy-girl ratio ranging from 4:1 to 6:1 (Cantwell, 1975b). Follow-up studies of these children indicate that they are prone to develop significant psychiatric and social problems in adolescence and later life. Antisocial behavior, serious academic retardation, poor self-image, and depression seem to be the most common outcomes in adolescence. Alcoholism, sociopathy, hysteria, and possible psychosis seem to be likely psychiatric outcomes in adulthood (Cantwell, 1975b).

The effectiveness of any drug treatment must thus be compared against the untreated natural history of the syndrome.

DIAGNOSTIC EVALUATION

No medication of any type should be instituted without a comprehensive diagnostic evaluation of the child. This should include: a detailed interview with the parents, a psychiatric evaluation of the child, information from the school, a physical and neurological examination, and appropriate laboratory studies

(Cantwell, 1975b). The interview with the parents and with the child have been described in detail elsewhere (Cantwell, 1975b).

The author recommends the use of the Rutter-Graham psychiatric rating scale for children. This scale rates specific items of behavior based on what the child has to say and on observation of the child during the interview. It has been shown to be a valid and reliable indicator of psychiatric illness in children (Rutter et al., 1970b). It should be recognized, however, that of all the elements that go into the evaluation, the interview with the child in a one-to-one setting may be the least favorable. It is very likely that the child who is described as hyperactive and distractible by parents and teachers will *not* appear so in a one-to-one setting.

Behavior rating scales completed by both parents and teachers should be obtained as baseline assessments of the child. The author recommends the Conners Parent Symptom Questionnaire, the Werry-Weiss-Peters Activity Scale, the Conners Teacher Questionnaire, and the Conners Abbreviated Symptom Questionnaire (Department of Health, Education and Welfare, 1973). The Conners Teacher Questionnaire has been shown to distinguish normal children from hyperactive children and to be quantitatively very sensitive to the behavioral effects of psychotropic drugs (Kupietz et al., 1972; Sprague et al., 1974; Sprague and Werry, 1974; Winsberg et al., 1972).

The Conners Parent Symptom Questionnaire, because it taps such a wide range of psychopathology, probably is not as useful in this group of children for assessing the effects of drug treatment as the Werry-Weiss-Peters Activity Scale (Werry and Sprague, 1970; Klein and Gittelman-Klein, 1975).

Ten items on the Conners Teacher Questionnaire and the Parent Symptom Questionnaire are identical and have been combined to form an Abbreviated Symptom Questionnaire which can be used by the physician to obtain frequent follow-up assessments of the child from both the parents and teachers. The abbreviated scale has been found to have almost the same sensitivity in obtaining statistically significant differences in psychotropic drug studies with hyperactive children (Sprague and Werry, 1974). For a further discussion of rating scales see Conners, ch. three.

A physical examination should always be done as part of the evaluation since in a minority of children defects of vision or hearing (Stewart et al., 1966) as well as abnormalities of speech (de Hirsch, 1973) may be identified. Baseline height and weight should be recorded in all children with frequent follow-up of these measures in children selected for stimulant drug therapy.

A careful pediatric neurologic examination should be part of the standard workup of every hyperactive child, if only to rule out a treatable or progressive neurologic disease. "Hard" evidence of neurological involvement is present in only a small minority of these children. Thus careful attention must be paid to the

detection of minor neurological abnormalities generally referred to in the literature as "soft" signs. Several good descriptions exist of developmental neurological examinations designed to elicit these minor neurological abnormalities
(Rutter et al., 1970a; Peters et al., 1973; Close, 1973; Werry et al., 1972). Goodman and Sours (1967) have described a play neurological examination which can
be done in conjunction with a psychiatric interview with the child. Evidence that
these minor neurologic abnormalities might be associated with a positive response to stimulant drug treatment will be discussed below.

Laboratory evaluations which might be considered in the workup of a child
with suspected minimal brain dysfunction include: clinical laboratory studies,
psychometric studies, and EEG. Neurophysiologic, chromosomal, metabolic,
and biochemical studies are only in the research realm at the present time. A
complete discussion of the utility of the various laboratory studies is beyond the
scope of this chapter and can be found elsewhere (Cantwell, 1975b).

A complete blood count and urinalysis should be done. In those children who
are placed on drug therapy certain other selected clinical laboratory studies
should be obtained at baseline and follow-up intervals (Cantwell, 1975b).

An EEG, in the author's opinion, need only be obtained when the history or
neurological examination suggests some definite neurological abnormality or
seizure disorder.

A psychoeducational assessment should be part of the workup of every child.
This evaluation should include, as a minimum, an assessment of general intelligence and academic achievement. Assessment of language functions, motor
functions, memory, and perception may be carried out as clinical needs indicate.
In this way any specific defects in intellectual, sensory, perceptual, or motor
functions can be detected (Cantwell, 1975b). Baseline evaluations of intellectual
ability and academic achievement also provide for some measure of long-term
gains in learning in those children on continuous drug treatment. The Wechsler
Intelligence Scale for Children (WISC), the Peabody Picture Vocabulary Test,
the Porteus Mazes, and the Peabody Individual Achievement Test are also useful
for this purpose.

CLINICAL MONITORING OF MEDICATION

Until there is a great deal of experimental evidence for the superiority of a new
drug, the author believes that a familiar and tested drug should be used as a first
choice. The initial amount should be the smallest available dose of the medica-

tion being used. A knowledge of the duration of action of the medication is necessary to determine optimal dose frequency for desired effect. Starting with a low dose the physician should increase the medication until either clinical improvement is noted or side effects occur which necessitate discontinuation of the drug. At present no laboratory or other measures exist by which medication can be titrated. The physician must use clinical judgement based on the information obtained from the parents, the school, and from direct observation of the child.

The instruments mentioned above, including both the Conners Parent and Teacher Rating Scales, as well as side-effect rating scales (Department of Health, Education and Welfare, 1973) can be used to assess systematically both the clinical effects and the side effects of the medication.

While there are *rough* guidelines for optimal dosage of individual drugs on a milligram of drug per kilogram of body weight basis, this is a controversial area. For example, Wender (1971) has advocated a high dose of 1.5 mg./kg. per day of dextroamphetamine and a high dose of 4.6 mg./kg. per day of methylphenidate.

Sprague and his colleagues have conducted laboratory studies showing that teacher ratings show an increased improvement in behavior ratings up to doses of .70 and 1.00 mg./kg. per day of methylphenidate. However this is double the dosage at which the peak enhancement of cognitive performance seems to occur (Sprague and Sleator, 1973).

It should be noted that an individual child may require a great deal more medication than would be expected on the basis of body weight, since large individual differences occur in blood levels of medication for comparable doses of the same drug in children of the same body weight. Also, a drug may have a therapeutic effect for a particular child only at a particular blood level. Children considered "nonresponders" to medication often simply have not been given an effective dose (Conners, 1972; Wender, 1971).

If improvement occurs, then seems to disappear, the dosage should be increased since tolerance to the effect of medication often develops (Arnold, 1973). As with amount of medication required, the development of tolerance is highly idiosyncratic. Some children remain on the same dosage of medication for a year or more and others develop tolerance much earlier.

The author recommends that all children should be given a drug-free trial at some time during the course of the extended medication treatment. There are several ways to do this. The best is to substitute placebo without letting the child or the schoolteacher know and determine by the rating scale if there is deterioration of behavior. However this method is not always available to the practicing physician.

Another way is to let the child go back to school in September without medication, and several weeks later obtain new ratings to compare with the rating obtained at the end of the previous school year when the child was on medication. If medication seems no longer required, the child should be followed closely to see if behavior deteriorates over time. Abstinence syndromes do not seem to develop during the drug-free trial.

At present no good way other than clinical judgement exists for determining when to discontinue medication. Medication should not be stopped because the child reaches a certain age, but only when the clinical picture indicates the child no longer requires it.

The physician must work closely with the child and parents in conjunction with the use of the medication. At the very least, the treating physician should help the child understand the nature of his difficulties and how the medication (and other therapeutic interventions) is intended to help the child help himself. The role and action of the medication in his life then can make more sense to the child and he will hopefully see the medication as one of *his* tools, not something forced on him by parents, teachers, or the doctor (Wender, 1971; Kehne, 1974).

The parents also should be prepared in a rational way for a trial of any medication. The physician should state that one medication may help a particular child but not help another, and that no sure way of predicting which medication might work for which child is yet available. The parents should also be told that the effective dose of a particular medication differs from one child to another.

For any particular drug used, the physician should explain in great detail to the parents what the expected benefits from the medication are and what the medication will *not* do. Expected side effects should also be discussed in detail and the parents encouraged to observe their child carefully for any likely side effects.

The time invested in this type of preparation of the child and his family will reap its benefits should the medication or the dosage have to be changed over a period of time in order to find the optimal dose of the optimal drug.

A most important (and often neglected) part of the physician's work in treating children with medication is establishing good rapport with the school. The child's teacher should be contacted either in person or by phone. Without cooperation from the school in reporting both positive and negative effects of the medication, it is impossible in the author's opinion to manage a child on any medication effectively. The teacher is likely to be the only person to see the child regularly in a group setting where he is required to do the same tasks as a large number of peers. Thus in a sense, the teacher is in a position to compare the performance of the index child with a "control group" on a daily basis.

This does not imply that the teacher controls either the prescribing or the regulation of medication, but that the physician needs to be in contact with the teacher in order to make the proper adjustments in the dosage of medication.

DRUG TREATMENT OF THE MINIMAL BRAIN
DYSFUNCTION SYNDROME

The decision to use one drug or another in the treatment of a child will ultimately be based on evidence in the literature for its effectiveness and safety. Difficulties in evaluating childhood psychopharmacologic studies arise from several sources: problems in classification and diagnosis, patient factors, family and environmental factors, drug factors, physician factors, and assessment techniques.

As discussed earlier, children with the "minimal brain dysfunction" syndrome form a clinically heterogenous group. In many studies no diagnostic criteria are specified and it is impossible to tell with what clinical picture the children presented. Thus other investigators cannot replicate the study and clinicians interested in treating children cannot tell what specific symptoms in which children were affected by the drug and which were not.

It is possible that children who are more severely ill and/or who have been ill for a longer period of time might not benefit as much from drug treatment as other children with the same behavioral picture but with a more acute or less severe course. However, severity and chronicity of the presenting clinical condition often are not reported.

Patient factors, including age, sex, I.Q., physical, and neurological findings are often not included as important variables. Thus populations of children reported in drug studies often include children of both sexes with a wide age and I.Q. range, despite evidence that each of these factors independently may play a role in response to drug treatment (Eisenberg & Conners, 1971). Likewise, certain physical and neurological factors likely to influence response to medication (Conners, 1971a) are often not evaluated or not reported.

Such familial and environmental considerations as social class, genetic factors, the presence or absence of parental psychopathology, and the parents' acceptance or rejection of drug treatment also are likely to affect drug response (Satterfield et al., 1973). Yet these are generally not taken into consideration.

Certain drug factors also are likely to affect response to treatment. (For example, whether the dosage in a study was fixed or whether the dosage was titrated against clinical symptoms.) Drug dosages are generally reported in total dosage per day rather than on a mg./kg. of body weight difference, even though the study sample may contain children with a wide range in age and body weight. Moreover, the amount of drug absorbed and ultimate blood level of the drug may be unequal for children of the same body weight receiving the same dose of medication. Very few studies report blood levels of medication.

Physician factors also play a role in treatment response. An enthusiastic, charismatic physician is likely to get a positive "placebo" response above and beyond whatever drug response is present. Very few drug studies take this into account.

And finally, the problems of assessment of drug effect must be considered. Judgments of effectiveness are influenced by whether molar aspects of behavior (evaluated by rating scales) or molecular aspects of behavior (usually rated by certain tests) (Conners, 1971a, and ch. three) are used to evaluate drug response. Since there are situational aspects of children's behavior, one should know whether the drug response is evaluated by the parents in the home, by teachers in the school, by laboratory investigation, or by physicians in the office. Teachers may report the drug as being effective in a classroom setting, yet no discernible change can be noted in the office or in a structured laboratory setting.

Finally, proper statistical analysis of any data obtained is vital for determination of effectiveness.

Very few if any drug studies control for all of these variables. Thus it is well for the clinician to keep in mind that conclusions about effectiveness or noneffectiveness of certain drugs may be based on data obtained from studies which did not take into account some of these key factors. With certain individual patients one or more of these factors may be of overriding importance in determining response to drug treatment.

SPECIFIC ASPECTS OF DRUG TREATMENT

Several critical reviews of the voluminous literature on drug treatment of the minimal brain dysfunction syndrome are available (Fish, 1968, 1975; Millichap and Fowler, 1967; Conners, 1970, 1971a, 1972; Werry and Sprague, 1972; Gittelman-Klein, 1975). Thus only selected aspects of clinical importance will be discussed here.

Central Nervous System Stimulants

Methylphenidate (Ritalin) and the amphetamines (dextroamphetamine, levo-amphetamine, and the racemic mixture), are the current drugs of choice in children with the minimal brain dysfunction syndrome. Improvement in behavior occurs in two-thirds to three-fourths of those children treated with these stimulants, while worsening can be expected in 5 to 10 percent (O'Malley and Eisenberg, 1973; Millichap, 1973; Cantwell, 1975b). Therapeutic properties and side effects are very similar. Both seem to act by potentiating norepinephrine and dopamine at central synapses (Ferris et al., 1972; Schildkraut and Kety, 1967).

The latency of onset of action for both stimulants is approximately thirty minutes with a three- to six-hour duration of action. Methylphenidate must be given at least twice a day to ensure an effective dose throughout the school day. The long-acting amphetamine spansules need be given only once a day.

The stimulants decrease hyperactivity and impulsivity and increase attention span. Total activity actually may be increased by the stimulants, crucial change being an increase in directed or contolled motor activity (Witt et al.; Millichap and Boldrey, 1967). The stimulants also produce small improvements in tests of general intelligence and visual motor perception and enhance performance in learning tasks (Knights and Hinton, 1969; Epstein et al., 1968; Werry et al., 1970; Conners et al., 1967). Breitmeyer (1969) suggested that stimulants produced a state-dependent learning effect in children; i.e., the children did not retain material they learned while on medication after the medication had been stopped. A series of studies from Sprague's laboratory (Sprague, 1972; Sprague and Werry, 1971), however, has failed to substantiate a state-dependency hypothesis.

Most children who respond to one stimulant will respond to the other, but some respond only to one (Conners, 1971b; Winsberg et al., 1974).

Anorexia, insomnia, headaches, stomachache, nausea, tearfulness, and pallor are common side effects with all the stimulants. In the author's experience the amphetamines, particularly dextroamphetamine, seem to produce more frequent and severe anorexia and insomnia.

While it is generally stated that stimulants do not produce euphoria in children, there has been very little systematic work on the effect of stimulant medication on mood. Long-term use of stimulants is known to produce depression in adults. This side effect is rarely mentioned in the literature on stimulant drug treatment of children (Ounsted, 1955). However the author has seen several children who developed mild to moderate depressive episodes in the course of treatment with both methylphenidate and amphetamine. These episodes required the cessation or reduction of dosage of the stimulant plus the use of imipramine, following which the depression lifted. Since depression in children may be difficult to detect, particularly in a child who was previously hyperactive, it should be looked for systematically in children receiving stimulant medication. Children who suddenly develop dysphoric mood whether constant, intermittent, or fluctuating, and who also present with a marked change in behavior, such as loss of self-confidence, withdrawal from social intercourse, school refusal, and somatic symptoms, should be suspected of having a mood disorder.

There does not seem to be a predilection for children who have been treated with stimulants to become drug abusers (Freedman, 1971; Beck et al., 1975). There is some suggestion that suppression of weight and height may occur with prolonged use of dextroamphetamine and suppression of weight, but not height, with methylphenidate (Safer and Allen, 1973; Safer et al., 1972). Effects on growth seem to be related to the anorexia caused by the medication. Children simply eat less while on the medication and return to previous growth patterns when taken off the drug (Safer and Allen, 1973; Safer et al., 1972; Schain and Reynard, 1975). Repeated measurements of height and weight of all children on stimulant medication should be charted on standard growth curves. When weight loss becomes a significant problem, some simple measures might be tried. The author recommends that the child eat a large breakfast prior to taking medication in the morning and/or a large supper when the effect of the medication has generally worn off. Also, if the child can be maintained off medication on the weekends and during the summer, appetite will usually improve, helping to alleviate some of the effects of decreased appetite which occur when the child is on medication. It is possible that appetite stimulants might be tried, but the author is unaware of any systematic studies in which this has been done.

Clinical experience suggests that most side effects of stimulant medication usually subside with time (Eisenberg, 1972); however, more systematic investigations of long-term effects of the use of stimulant medication are still needed.

Other stimulants, in addition to methylphenidate and the amphetamines, have been tried in children with minimal brain dysfunction. These include: magnesium pemoline (Cylert), deanol (Deanor) and caffeine.

Magnesium pemoline is a weak central nervous system stimulant which has the claimed advantage of long duration of action so that one daily dose is sufficient. Preliminary results indicate that it is about as effective as the amphetamines in the treatment of children with minimal brain dysfunction, but no more so (Conners et al., 1972; Page et al., 1972). There is evidence that magnesium pemoline takes longer to induce a significant clinical effect than the amphetamines (Conners et al., 1972).

Deanol also acts as a central nervous system stimulant, possibly by conversion to acetylcholine within neurons. A recent review of the literature indicated that better-controlled studies with deanol tended to show little or no drug effect and it is no longer considered to have any value in the treatment of minimal brain dysfunction in children (Conners, 1973).

Coffee, with caffeine the presumed active ingredient, has been reported to be as effective as methylphenidate in one study (Schnackenberg, 1973). Preliminary results of well-controlled studies using caffeine tablets do not substantiate this finding (Conners, 1975; Garfinkel et al., 1975; Arnold, 1974).

The side effects of these central nervous system stimulants are similar to those of methylphenidate and the amphetamines.

Tricyclic Antidepressants

The role of tricyclic antidepressants in the treatment of minimal brain dysfunction is controversial. Investigators have found imipramine (Tofranil) to be effective in 40 to 85 percent of children with minimal brain dysfunction (Huessy and Wright, 1970; Winsberg et al., 1972; Waizer et al., 1974; Rapoport et al., 1974). The mean dosage in these studies ranged from 50–175 mg. per day and this could explain the reported range in effectiveness. However, the mean dosage in the Huessy and Wright study was only 50 mg. per day, with a single bedtime dose providing a therapeutic effect evident the next day. This is distinctly different from the antidepressant effect of these medications, which takes from two to three weeks to occur. The nighttime dosage schedule offers a distinct advantage if future studies support the efficacy of imipramine, but there is some indication that the likelihood of toxicity from imipramine is increased by a single dose at nighttime (Winsberg et al., in press).

The main side effects of imipramine include anorexia, nausea, weight loss, insomnia, dry mouth, drowsiness, dizziness, and gastric upset. Some investigators reported that a rapid withdrawal of imipramine leads to severe nausea and vomiting (Katz et al., 1975). Despite the promising results of some of the above studies, other investigators in this field found that while imipramine may initially control hyperactivity, the children's behavior deteriorates over a two- to three-month period (Katz et al., 1975). As of yet, imipramine is not approved by the FDA for use with children under the age of twelve except for enuresis. Moreover, as a result of recent reports of EKG abnormalities in children treated with imipramine (Winsberg et al., 1975), the FDA has decided to approve investigational protocols for the use of imipramine only for certain dose ranges for children of specified body weights, and regular EKG monitoring is recommended (Hayes et al., 1975).

Major Tranquilizers

The rather extensive literature on the use of the major tranquilizers consists of mostly uncontrolled studies and contradictory findings (Freeman, 1970; Sprague and Werry, 1971). Thioridazine (Mellaril) and chlorpromazine (Thorazine) seem to be the most frequently used phenothiazines. Certainly their effects are not as well documented as those of the stimulants. Some investigators (Cytryn et al., 1960) failed to observe improvement, while others reported that chlorpromazine decreased hyperactivity, but not distractibility (Weiss et al., 1968). Moreover, the type of improvement obtained with chlorpromazine was not as satisfactory as that obtained with stimulant medication (Weiss et al., 1971b).

Some clinicians (Winsberg et al., in press) found chlorpromazine and thiorodazine to be equally effective with dosages beginning at 25 mg. three times a day with increments up to a maximum dosage of 150–200 mg. per day. Most common side effects included sedation, extrapyramidal, and dystonic reactions; and anticholinergic symptoms, including constipation, dry mouth, and blurred vision. Side effects reported with long-term use of phenothiazines include tardive dyskinesia and seizures (Winsberg et al., in press).

However, others found the phenothiazines to be much less satisfactory to use than the stimulants (Katz et al., 1975). Few children could be maintained on thioridazine alone and significant improvement in social and academic areas was not comparable to that found with stimulant medication. Side effects were frequent at higher doses.

There is general agreement that major tranquilizers produce deleterious effects on learning and cognitive functioning (Hartlage, 1965; Conners, 1971a). In addition, maintenance over a long period of time on the phenothiazines has been reported to cause a gradual deterioration in behavior and mood of the children. This occurs even after an initial positive response to the medication.

In summary, phenothiazines may be indicated and more effective than stimulants for certain individual children. However, they are not the drugs of first choice. The evidence for their efficacy is not nearly as well documented as that of the stimulants and their potential toxicity is greater (Conners, 1972; Katz et al., 1975).

The major tranquilizer Haloperidol (Haldol), a butyrophenone, deserves mention. Several studies (Cunningham et al., 1968; Barker and Fraser, 1968; Wong and Cock, 1971; LeVann, 1971) indicate that motor activity, restlessness, aggressive behavior, and impulsive behavior are target symptoms significantly affected by Haldol. It is not a drug of first choice, however, for children with minimal brain dysfunction. It is generally felt to be most effective when organic factors play a role in the etiology of the child's disorder (Barker, 1975). Dosage of Haldol ranges from .05 to 0.1 mg./kg. of body weight for twenty-four hours given in two divided doses. Side effects and toxic effects include: drowsiness, which is generally transient, and dystonic reactions, which occur with higher dosage. The latter are more common in older children. Parkinsonian signs may also occur with high dosages. Some investigators (Polizos et al., 1973) have mentioned withdrawal effects. Long-term use apparently does not result in significant adverse effects.

Lithium Carbonate

Lithium carbonate has been tried with varying success by several investigators (Whitehead and Clark, 1970; Greenhill et al., 1973). It is not as effective as the stimulants in treatment of the usual child. In the extremely rare case of mania presenting with hyperactivity in the prepubertal child, lithium carbonate may be the treatment of choice. Since blood levels of lithium are rather easily monitored, side effects and toxic effects can be kept to a minimum.

Antihistamines

Although the antihistamine diphenhydramine (Benadryl) has been advocated by some, probably because of its sedative effect, the efficacy of this medication with MBD children has not yet been proved in a comparative trial using objective measures of evaluation (Fish, 1975).

Other Psychopharmacologic Agents

There is general agreement that sedatives such as phenobarbital are usually contraindicated for children with minimal brain dysfunction (Conners, 1972).

In contrast to their very common use with adults, the minor tranquilizers, especially the benzodiazipines are rather infrequently used for children with minimal brain dysfunction. Although there are a few studies that show them to be somewhat effective (Millichap, 1973), by and large these are generally uncontrolled studies using nonobjective measures of improvement. In the author's experience these agents have been relatively ineffective, whether alone or in combination with other medication in treating the usual MBD child.

Drug Combinations

Generally the author believes that use of a single medication for a child with minimal brain dysfunction is preferable to the use of multiple medications. Particularly deplored are the use of "drug cocktails" with mixtures of three or more medications. In these cases the author believes that side effects are much more likely to become additive than are clinical effects. Moreover, it becomes almost impossible to assess what medication is affecting (or producing) what symptoms.

There are some combinations of drugs which may be useful in individual cases, although the author feels that they form a small proportion of the total cases treated.

The first two combinations include a stimulant plus an antihistamine or a stimulant plus a phenothiazine. Both of these combinations are useful for children who respond nicely to a stimulant medication, but who have severe sleep problems. In these cases the use of either an antihistamine (such as Benadryl) or phenothiazine (such as Mellaril or Thorazine) has been found to be effective in treating the sleep difficulty.

The combination of a stimulant plus a phenothiazine has also been found to be effective in those children who have responded to the stimulants clinically, but in whom side effects preclude further increase of stimulant medication. In these cases, and in cases where the stimulant medication produces an "up and down effect'' as the medication wears off, the added effect of a more stable, long-acting phenothiazine may be quite beneficial.

The third combination of a stimulant plus a tricyclic antidepressant has only rarely been used by the author. These have been in cases where depression appeared as a side effect in those children who had been successfully treated with a stimulant medication. Some of these cases required the cessation of the stimulant medication, but in other cases a moderate dose of the tricyclic (such as 50 mg. of Tofranil at bedtime) has been found to alleviate completely the depression. It should be recognized that the stimulant medication probably increases the blood level of the tricyclic so that the dosage level would be expected to be lower than that used to treat a primary affective disorder. Other investigators (Katz et al., 1975) have found this combination to be useful for those children who respond to a stimulant medication, but develop separation anxiety during the course of treatment.

LONG-TERM EFFECTS OF MEDICATION

There is very limited evidence available on the long-term effect of any medication on children with minimal brain dysfunction. In a five-year follow-up of hyperactive children (Weiss et al., 1971a; Minde et al., 1971; Minde et al., 1972) the Montreal group reported that sixty-six of the children had received chlorpromazine up to 200 mg. daily while thirty-eight had dextroamphetamine up to 20 mg. daily following their initial evaluation. Thirty-two had taken medication less than six months, thirty-seven remained on medication between one and three years, and twenty-two had taken it for three years or more. Only twelve were still taking any medication at the time of follow-up. Forty-six had discontinued medication because it was ineffective or because of side effects and only fourteen because sufficient improvement had occurred. There was no significant correlation between psychological adjustment and length of time the patients had been maintained on medication. In fact, there was a trend for those on medication the longest period of time to be more poorly adjusted at follow-up.

Mendelson et al. (1971) followed up a group of hyperactive children from the St. Louis Children's Hospital. Forty percent were still in treatment at the time of follow-up at the Children's Hospital and another 14 percent were in treatment elsewhere. Ninety-two percent had received stimulant medication, coupled in some cases with supportive psychotherapy for the children and counseling for the parents. Sixty percent of the children were reported as improved for at least six months while on stimulants, 12 percent had deteriorated and the outcome was equivocal in 28 percent.

Quinn and Rapoport (1975) in a one-year follow-up study of seventy-six hyperkinetic boys who had been treated with either methylphenidate or imipramine found that those who were still on treatment at the time of follow-up were rated significantly better by their teachers than the group receiving no treatment at follow-up. However, the parents rated those children receiving no treatment equal to those children receiving either methylphenidate or imipramine in terms of behavior at the time of follow-up. More children who had been treated with imipramine discontinued the medication during the course of the year (nineteen out of thirty-seven) than did children taking methylphenidate (nine out of thirty-eight).

The most disappointing results of long-term drug treatment of hyperactive children were obtained by Weiss et al. (1975). They compared three groups of children five years after initial evaluation. Twenty-two of the children had taken chlorpromazine for eighteen months to five years and two children were still taking the medication at the time of follow-up. Twenty-four children had taken methylphenidate from three to five years during the period of evaluation and twelve were still taking the medication at the time of follow-up. The control group was twenty children who had received no drug treatment at all. The results indicated that although the hyperactivity scores decreased significantly in all three groups, there were no significant differences between the three groups of children. There were also no differences between the groups in delinquency, emotional adjustment, academic performance (as measured by the number of grades failed), and in performance on certain psychological tests, including the Wechsler Intelligence Test for Children and the Bender-Gestalt. The authors point out that the measures of outcome used were very gross and that clinical observations at the time of follow-up indicated that methylphenidate did help the children, both at home and at school. However, it apparently had no significant effect upon long-term outcome, at least by the measures that were used by the authors. It also is not clear from their paper whether all of the children were intensively and consistently treated by the same people throughout the time of the follow-up.

In summary, none of the studies has clearly demonstrated that drug treatment significantly alters the long-term prognosis of children with minimal brain dysfunction. But it must be stated that a definitive study has not yet been carried out.

PREDICTORS OF TREATMENT RESPONSE

Little is known about the predictors of treatment response. In one of the few attempts to discover clinical predictors, Barcai (1971) found both the clinical interview and a "finger twitch" test to be useful in differentiating responders to amphetamine from nonresponders. With the child sitting opposite the examiner, hands hung between his knees in a normal position, the fingers moderately flexed, the interval between the start of the test and the time of the first twitch of a hand or finger was recorded. The finger twitch appeared in all nonresponders after twenty-five seconds and eighteen of twenty-one positive or equivocal responders before twenty-five seconds elapsed.

The items from the clinical interview with the child found to be most helpful in differentiating responders from nonresponders were the presence in the drug responders of: excess body movements, poor language ability, lack of ability to abstract and to use imagination constructively, lack of adjustment to the values of society, and lack of planning ability.

Satterfield (1973a) found that older children had a better response to methylphenidate, as did children who had more behavioral abnormalities reported by the teacher. In contrast, other investigators found that severity of symptoms and general psychiatric status were not related to drug response (Cytryn et al., 1960).

Some investigators have felt that markedly antisocial children who may be rated as hyperactive by teachers are unlikely to respond to psychopharmacologic management (Katz et al., 1975).

The presence of "organic factors" has been claimed by a number of authors to predict a good response to stimulant treatment, but the findings have not been consistent (Pincus and Glaser, 1966; Zrull et al., 1966; Epstein et al., 1968; Conrad and Insel, 1967; Satterfield, 1973a and b; Millichap, et al., 1968; Werry et al., 1966; Burks, 1964; Steinberg et al., 1971). However, the indicators of organicity in the different studies are not the same and it is difficult to compare results.

Steinberg (1971) found that children with "soft" neurologic signs were more likely to respond to dextroamphetamine. Satterfield (1973b) found that children with soft neurological signs and children with abnormal EEGs were both independently likely to respond to methylphenidate treatment. Those children who had both soft neurological signs and an abnormal EEG were the most likely to respond. However, Werry et al. (1966) found that the presence of an EEG abnormality was unrelated to response to chlorpromazine. Conrad and Insel (1967) found that children who were considered to be "organic" on the basis of historical data were more likely to respond to amphetamine. The findings of Epstein et al. (1968) are consistent with Conrad and Insel's.

Thus, while there is some indication that MBD children with demonstrable neurological dysfunction may be more likely to respond to stimulant drug treatment, the evidence to date is not conclusive. Most of these studies have also shown that many MBD children respond to stimulant drug treatment even in the absence of any indicators of organicity (Conners, 1966; Gittelman-Klein, 1975).

In a series of studies, Satterfield and his associates (Satterfield et al., 1974) found six neurophysiological predictors of response to methylphenidate: low skin conductance level, high amplitude EEG, high energy in the low-frequency band of the EEG, large amplitude evoked cortical response and slow recovery of the evoked response. These measures are consistent with the hypothesis that the pathophysiology of some children with the syndrome is low central nervous system arousal level. According to this hypothesis, the low arousal leads to insufficient cortical inhibitory control over both sensory input and motor functions. The stimulants then act by stimulating the mid-brain reticular activating system (Killam, 1968) resulting in a net increase of cortical inhibitory control over both sensory and motor functions. This increased control over motor functions enables the child to reduce nongoal-directed inappropriate motor behavior. The increased inhibitory control over sensory input should enable the child to inhibit nonmeaningful stimuli in order to attend selectively in a learning situation.

That stimulant medication does result in increased cortical inhibitory control over sensory functions is suggested not only by improvement in behavior, but also from electrophysiological studies. Satterfield et al. (1974) found a decrease in evoked response to nonmeaningful auditory stimuli in those children who responded positively to methylphenidate treatment. Several studies have reported increased habituation of peripheral responsivity to stimuli following administration of stimulant medication to hyperkinetic children. Conners (1971b) found that dextroamphetamine enhanced the rate of habituation of finger blood volume response to auditory stimuli. Similar results have been reported for heart rate and galvanic skin response following methylphenidate (Conners, 1971b).

Also consistent with the hypothesis of increased inhibitory functions are Laufer's finding of an increased photometrazol threshold (Laufer et al., 1957) and Shetty's finding of an increased amount of alpha rhythm (1971) following the administration of dextroamphetamine to hyperkinetic children. However, there are also neurophysiological studies which are not consistent with the hypothesis of low central nervous system arousal (Montagu, 1975).

Wender (1971) proposed that MBD children have an abnormality in the metabolism of the central neurotransmitters: serotonin, norepinephrine, and dopamine. He felt that the biochemical abnormality affects the behavior of these children by impairing the reward mechanism in the activating system of the brain. He hypothesized that these children have a diminished capacity for positive and negative affect which he termed "anhedonia." The differential effect of the isomers of amphetamine, levoamphetamine, and dextroamphetamine, on the behavior of MBD children (Arnold et al., 1973) offered indirect evidence that in some children the disorder is mediated by dopaminergic systems and in others by norepinephrinergic systems.

More direct studies of a possible metabolic abnormality have been limited.

Wender et al. (1971) failed to detect any differences in the metabolites of sero-tonin, norepinephrine, or dopamine in the urine of MBD children compared to a group of normal children. However the study population was very heterogenous. Wender (1969) did find very low concentrations of serotonin in the blood plate-lets of three hyperactive children, all of whom were from the same family. In the rest of the study population, the platelet serotonin levels were normal or in the borderline range. Coleman (1971) demonstrated low platelet serotonin concen-trations in 88 percent of twenty-five hyperactive children. The two most hyperac-tive children in the group were studied in a research ward. Interestingly, the sero-tonin concentration rose toward the normal range and the hyperactivity of the children lessened during the hospital stay. When both children returned home the serotonin values dropped to prehospitalization levels and hyperactivity in-creased. Urinary monoamine metabolites in both of these children remained within normal limits during their hospital stay.

Rapoport et al. (1970) found an inverse relationship between the degree of hyperactive behavior and urinary norepinephrine excretion within a group of hyperactive boys, but the mean twenty-four-hour urinary catecholamines excre-tion did not differentiate the patient group from a normal comparison group. In addition there was an inverse relationship between response of the hyper-activity to dextroamphetamine and urinary norepinephrine levels.

Satterfield (1973a) found that drug response was unrelated to the presence of psychopathology in either first- or second-degree relatives in the family. Conrad and Insel (1967) found that children whose parents were rated as "grossly de-viant" or "socially incompetent" were less likely to respond positively to medi-cation, even in the face of other factors which tended to predict a good response.

Studies of family interaction in relation to drug response have been limited and inconsistent. The Montreal group (Weiss et al., 1968; Werry et al., 1966) found that the mother-child relationship and the quality of the home were unrelated to drug therapy, but in a later study (Weiss et al., 1971b) there was a positive asso-ciation between response to methylphenidate and the quality of the mother-child relationship. Other authors (Knobel, 1962; Kraft, 1968) have noted that the atti-tude of the family to the child's taking medication is likely to affect treatment response. However, few studies have attempted to look at family variables in a systematic way.

More systematic research in this area is sorely needed, with careful comprehen-sive consideration of stimulus factors, response parameters, sociofamilial and organismic factors that might be related to treatment response (Conners, 1972).

DRUG THERAPY COMBINED WITH OTHER
THERAPEUTIC INTERVENTIONS

In concluding this chapter it is well to emphasize that for management purposes a child with minimal brain dysfunction is best considered a multi-handicapped child requiring a multiple modality treatment approach (Cantwell, 1975b). Any or all of the intervention approaches discussed below may be necessary for an individual child. Treatment must be individualized and based on a comprehensive assessment of each child and his family.

There are very few systematic studies of other treatment modalities used in children with minimal brain dysfunction and there are even fewer studies of drug therapy used in combination with other therapies. Too often drug treatment is viewed as an "either/or proposition"; i.e., either drugs are used or some other modality. However, in the usual case drugs will have to be used in combination with other modalities, based on an individual assessment of each child and his family.

Individual Psychotherapy with the Child

As with the other psychiatric disorders of childhood (Levitt, 1957, 1963; Rachman, 1971) evidence for the efficacy of individual psychotherapy for children with minimal brain dysfunction is lacking (Cytryn et al., 1960). However, psychotherapy is indicated for the secondary emotional symptoms of depression, low self-esteem and poor peer relationships. Gardner (1973) has described the active and innovative techniques he has found useful in treating the secondary complications of children with minimal brain dysfunction. However, to date the author is unaware of any systematic, long-term comparisons made of children treated with medication plus psychotherapy to children treated with medication alone. This is a crucial area for future research.

Behavior Modification

Until recently studies of MBD children using operant conditioning techniques have been limited to single cases (Patterson et al., 1965; Ward, 1966) or to very small numbers of children (Doubros and Daniels, 1966; Sprague, 1973). In a direct comparison of behavioral and drug treatment, Christensen and Sprague (1973) compared six children receiving placebo and behavior modification with six children receiving methylphenidate and behavior modification. Using seat activity and daily quizzes as outcome measures, the investigators found that the drug-plus-behavior-modification group had significantly lower seat activity than the placebo-plus-behavior-modification group, but there were no significant differences between the groups on number of correct answers in the daily quizzes.

In a similar study Christensen (1973) found a number of significant differences between groups on a variety of measures including: Conners Teacher Rating Scale, the Werry-Quay Observational Measures, productivity and accuracy of academic materials, and seat activity. The behavior-modification procedure alone accounted for most of the significant improvements over baseline recordings. Methylphenidate was not found to be consistently superior to behavior modification alone on any measure. This latter study, however, was conducted with institutionalized mentally retarded hyperkinetic children and the results may not be generalized to other children with the syndrome.

In the best direct comparative study of behavior modification and medication, Gittelman-Klein et al. (1975) set out to investigate the relative merits of behavior therapy, a combination of behavior therapy and methylphenidate, and methylphenidate alone in a group of hyperkinetic children. Their preliminary report included a study of twenty-two children, of whom six had received behavior therapy and placebo, eight behavior therapy and methylphenidate, and six methylphenidate alone. On the Conners Teacher Rating Scale there was a significant advantage for children receiving methylphenidate as opposed to those receiving behavior therapy alone, on both the "Hyperactivity" and the "Conduct" factors. There was no significant difference between those children receiving behavior therapy and methylphenidate and those receiving methylphenidate alone.

Similar results were obtained with other measures used in the study. The authors are quick to point out that the results presented to date are based on very small sample sizes. However, should the results continue with a larger sample size, certain trends present in the data now indicating superiority of medication over behavior therapy will become consistently significant.

Further research is needed in this area with larger numbers of children over longer periods of follow-up and using multiple measures of outcome, particularly measures of academic performance.

Educational Management

Each year a child spends about 1400 hours out of 8716 waking hours in school (McCarthy, 1973). Thus it is important that teachers be as familiar as parents with the syndrome and there must be consistency of expectations and methods of behavior reinforcement between the home and the school. Most MBD children can tolerate and will need to remain in a regular classroom. However, for those children with significant learning disabilities specific remediation procedures based on a thorough psychoeducational assessment are a necessity. However, there is little hard evidence to support the efficacy of most special education programs (Dunn, 1968; Haywood, 1966).

Well-controlled studies of special education programs are few in number and disappointing in results. Conrad et al. (1971) randomly assigned sixty-eight hyperkinetic children matched for intelligence and degree of hyperactivity to one of four experimental groups: placebo/no tutoring; placebo/tutoring; dextroamphetamine/no tutoring; dextroamphetamine/tutoring. The tutoring alone produced little benefit, while those who received both tutoring and dextroamphetamine showed improvement in behavior and on a number of psychological tests. However, the dextroamphetamine only group showed the most improvement. Most disappointing was the fact that only three of the sixty-eight children made enough progress in the year of the study to no longer need remedial help.

While it is unrealistic to expect the child who is two or three grade levels behind at the time that he is initially seen to suddenly make up those two to three years with the addition of any medication, it must be said that there is no hard evidence as yet that special education programs for children with minimal brain dysfunction have any long-term efficacy. Moreover, the availability of such individualized special training in the public school system is limited at best.

Family Involvement

The author believes that successful management of the minimal brain dysfunction syndrome requires the involvement of the entire family. The use of parent groups modeled after those described by Patterson (1971) has been found to be an effective treatment modality, in the absence of severe psychopathology in the parents. In these groups the parents are taught the nature and phenomenology of the syndrome, the basics of social learning theory and behavior modification, and the principles of structuring their child's environment so that there are regular daily routines and firm limits on his behavior. The importance of avoiding situations known to cause difficulty, overstimulation, and excessive fatigue are emphasized. Videotaping segments of parent-child interaction and playing back the maladaptive behaviors with explicit instructions to the parents on how to deal with them has been found to be helpful (Feighner, 1975).

The use of two group leaders, each with different roles, has been found by the author to be quite helpful. One group leader concentrates on more dynamic and interpersonal issues for about one-half of the group session, and in the other half of the session the other group leader concentrates on the parent training. The group format allows the parents to give each other mutual support and also provides for an exchange of information regarding community resources, school funding, parent organizations, and other issues.

The use of siblings in the planning and carrying out of behavioral programs in the homes is a promising new technique (Miller and Cantwell, 1975). It can reasonably be assumed that siblings do influence each other because of the amount of time and space they share and because of the intense long-term relationships that siblings are required to have with each other. However, there has been little systematic effort to analyze sibling interaction or to make use of them as change agents. Those programs that have used siblings as surrogate therapists have been found to be quite effective in: teaching MBD children new skills, helping to provide a consistent predictable environment, helping the child to produce desirable behavior and decrease maladaptive behavior, and carrying out programs when parents are not available either physically or emotionally (Miller and Cantwell, 1975). In two separate research studies the author has seen demonstrated improvement in both parent and teacher ratings of behavior above and beyond that obtained by drug treatment alone after direct family-intervention programs using siblings as surrogate therapists have been introduced.

Other Therapeutic Modalities

There are a variety of other therapeutic modalities that have been advocated by certain individuals for children with minimal brain dysfunction. Among these are neurophysiological retraining such as patterning, optometry, and sensory integrative therapy (Silver, 1975).

Megavitamin therapy, elimination diets, and hypoglycemic diets have also been touted (Cantwell, 1975b; Silver, 1975). In the author's opinion there is no hard scientific evidence for the efficacy of any of these therapies used individually. Moreover, there is no good comparative study of these therapies versus drug therapy or in combination with drug therapy.

SUMMARY

A critical review of the literature dealing with treatment of the child with minimal brain dysfunction reveals the following:

1. Central nervous system stimulants are effective for some symptoms of some children over the short haul. Methylphenidate and the amphetamines seem to be the drugs of choice.

2. Other drugs in general have not been found to be as effective as the central nervous system stimulants.

3. Little is known about how to predict whether an *individual* child will respond to a particular drug. However, several studies of *groups* of children indicate that there are neurological, neurophysiological, familial, environmental, and clinical factors that are important predictors of response.

4. More information is needed about the long-term efficacy and safety of the medications currently used to treat MBD children.

5. Studies of other treatment modalities used with MBD children are fewer in

number than reports of drug studies and little is known about their long-term effects.

6. Even less is known about the combination of drug treatment plus other treatment modalities particularly over the long haul.

7. Involvement of the family is critical to the success of any management program, but familial factors are rarely mentioned in studies of treatment.

8. Successful management of an individual child will involve the use of multiple treatment approaches.

References

Arnold, L. (1973), The art of medicating hyperkinetic children: A number of practical suggestions. *Clin. Ped., 12,* 135–41.

Arnold, L. (1974), Personal communication.

Barcai, A. (1971), Predicting the response of children with learning disabilities and behavior problems to dextroamphetamine sulfate: The clinical interview and the finger twitch test. *Pediatrics, 47,* 73–80.

Barker, P. (1975), Haloperidol. *J. Ch. Psych. and Psychiat., 16,* 169–172.

Barker, P., and Fraser, I. A. (1968), A controlled trial of haloperidol in children. *Brit. J. Psychiat., 114,* 855–857.

Beck, L., Langford, W., MacKay, M., and Sum, G. (1975), Childhood chemotherapy and later drug abuse and growth curve: A follow-up study of 30 adolescents. *Am. J. Psychiat., 132,* 436–438.

Breitmeyer, J. M. (1969), *Effects of thioridazine and methylphenidate on learning retention in retardates.* Unpublished master's thesis, Univ. of Ill.

Burks, H. F. (1964), Effects of amphetamine therapy on hyperkinetic children. *Arch. Gen. Psychiat., 11,* 604–609.

Cantwell, D. P. (1972), Psychiatric illness in families of hyperactive children. *Arch. Gen. Psychiat., 27,* 414–417.

Cantwell, D. P. (1975a), Genetic studies of hyperactive children: Psychiatric illness in biologic and adopting parents. In R. Fieve, D. Rosenthall, and H. Brill (Eds.), *Genetic research in psychiatry.* Baltimore: Johns Hopkins University Press, 273–280.

Cantwell, D. P. (1975b), *The hyperactive child: Diagnosis, management and current research.* New York: Spectrum Publications.

Cantwell, D. P. (in press), The hyperkinetic syndrome. In M. Rutter, and H. Hersov (Eds.), *Recent advances in child psychiatry.* London: Blackwell.

Christensen, D. (1973), *The combined effects of methylphenidate (Ritalin) and a classroom behavior modification program in reducing the hyperkinetic behavior of institutionalized mental retardates.* Unpublished doctoral dissertation, Univ. of Ill.

Christensen, D., and Sprague, R. (1973), Reduction of hyperactive behavior by conditioning procedures alone and combined with methylphenidate (Ritalin). *Behavior Res. Ther., 11,* 331–334.

Clements, S. (1966), *Minimal brain dysfunction in children.* NINDB Monograph No. 3. Washington, D.C.: U.S. Public Health Service.

Close, J. (1973), Scored neurological examination. *Psychopharm. Bull.,* DHEW, pp. 142–50.

Coleman, M. (1971), Serotonin concentrations in whole blood of hyperactive children. *J. Ped., 73,* 985–990.

Conners, C. K. (1966), The effect of Dexedrine on rapid discrimination and motor control of hyperkinetic children under mild stress. *J. Nerv. Ment. Dis., 142,* 429–433.

Conners, C. K. (1970), The use of stimulant drugs in enhancing performance learning. In W. L. Smith, (Ed.), *Drugs and cerebral function.* Springfield: Charles C. Thomas, pp. 85–98.

Conners, C. K. (1971a), Drugs in the management of children with learning disabilities. In L. Tarnopol (Ed.), *Learning disorders in children: Diagnosis, medication, education*. Boston: Little, Brown and Co. pp. 253–302.

Conners, C. K. (1971b), Recent drug studies with hyperkinetic children. *J. Learn. Disabil., 4*, 476–483.

Conners, C. K. (1972), Pharmacotherapy of psychopathology in children. In H. Quay, and J. Werry (Eds.), *Psychopathological disorders of childhood*. New York: Wiley and Sons, pp. 316–348.

Conners, C. K. (1973), Deanol and behavior disorders in children: A critical review of the literature and recommended future studies for determining efficacy. *Psychopharma. Bull.*, DHEW, pp. 188–195.

Conners, C. K. (1975), A placebo-crossover study of caffeine treatment of hyperkinetic children. *Int. J. Ment. Health, 4*, 132–143.

Conners, C. K., Eisenberg, L., and Barcai, A. (1967), Effect of dextroamphetamine on children. *Arch. Gen. Psychiat., 17*, 478–485.

Conners, C. K., Taylor, E., Meo, G., Kurtz, M., and Fournier, M. (1972), Magnesium pemoline and dextroamphetamine: A controlled study in children with minimal brain dysfunction. *Psychopharmacologica, 26*, 321–36.

Conrad, W., and Insel, J. (1967), Anticipating the response to amphetamine therapy in the treatment of hyperkinetic children. *Pediatrics, 40*, 96–99.

Conrad, W., Dworkin E., Shai, A., and Tobiessen, J. (1971), Effects of amphetamine therapy and prescriptive tutoring on the behavior and achievement of lower class hyperactive children. *J. Learn. Dis., 4*, 509–517.

Cunningham, M. A., Pillai, V., and Rogers, W. J. B. (1968), Haloperidol in the treatment of children with severe behavior disorders. *Brit. J. Psychiat., 114*, 845–854.

Cytryn, L., Gilbert, A., and Eisenberg, L. (1960), The effectiveness of tranquilizing drugs plus supportive psychotherapy in treating behavior disorders of children: A double-blind study of eighty outpatients. *Am. J. Orthopsychiat., 30*, 113–128.

de Hirsch, K. (1973), Early language development and minimal brain dysfunction. *Ann. N.Y. Acad. Sci., 205*, 158–163.

Doubros, S., and Daniels, G. (1966), An experimental approach to the reduction of overactive behavior. *Behaviour Res. Ther., 4*, 251–258.

Dunn, L. M. (1968), Special education for the mildly retarded—is much of it justifiable? *Exceptional Children, 35*, 5–22.

Eisenberg, L. (1972), The hyperkinetic child and stimulant drugs. *New Eng. J. Med., 287*, 249–50.

Eisenberg, L., and Conners, C. K. (1971), Psychopharmacology in childhood. In N. Talbot, J. Kagan, and L. Eisenberg (Eds.), *Behavioral science in pediatric medicine*. Philadelphia: W. B. Saunders Co., pp. 397–423.

Epstein, L., Lasagna, L., Conners, C., and Rodriguez, A. (1968), Correlation of dextroamphetamine excretion and drug response in hyperkinetic children. *J. Nerv. Ment. Dis., 146*, 136–146.

Feighner, A. (1975), Videotape training for parents as therapeutic agents with hyperactive children. In D. Cantwell (Ed.), *The hyperactive child: Diagnosis, management and current research*. New York: Spectrum Publications, pp. 145–157.

Ferris, R. M., Tang, F. L. M., and Maxwell, R. A. (1972), A comparison of the capacities of isomers of amphetamine deoxypipradol and methylphenidate to inhibit the uptake of tritiated catecholamines into rat cerebral cortex slices, synaptosomal preparations of rat cerebral cortex, hypothalamus and striatum into adrenergic nerves of rabbit aorta. *J. Pharm. and Exp. Ther., 181*, 407–416.

Fish, B. (1968), Methodology in child psychopharmacology. In D. Efron (Ed.), *Psychopharmacology, review of progress, 1957–1967*, Washington D.C.: Public Health Service Publication No. 1836, pp. 989–1001.

Fish, B. (1975), Drug treatment of the hyperactive child. In D. Cantwell (Ed.), *The hyperactive child: Diagnosis, management and current research*. New York: Spectrum Publications, pp. 109–127.

Freedman, D. (1971), Report on the conference on the use of stimulant drugs in the treatment of behaviorally disturbed young school children. *Psychopharma. Bull., 7*, 23.

Freeman, R. (1970), Psychopharmacology and the retarded child. In F. Menolascino (Ed.), *Psychiatric approaches to mental retardation*. New York: Basic Books, pp. 294–368.

Gardner, R. A. (1973), Psychotherapy of the psychogenic problems secondary to minimal brain dysfunction. *Int. J. Ch. Psychother., 2*, 224–256.

Garfinkel, B., Webster, C., and Sloman, L. (1975), Methylphenidate and caffeine in the treatment of children with minimal brain dysfunction. *Am. J. Psychiat., 132,* 723–728.

Gesell, A., and Amatruda, C. S. (1949), *Developmental diagnosis,* 2nd Ed. New York: Hoeber.

Gittelman-Klein, R. (1975), Review of clinical psychopharmacological treatment of hyperkinesis. In D. Klein, and R. Gittelman-Klein (Eds.), *Progress in psychiatric drug treatment.* New York: Bruner/Mazel, pp. 661–674.

Gittelman-Klein, R., Klein, D. F., Abikoff, H., Felixbrod, J., Katz, S., Gloisten, A., Kates, W., and Saraf, K. (1975), Presented at the 128th Annual Meeting of American Psychiatric Association, Anaheim, Ca., May 5–9, 1975.

Goodman, J., and Sours, J. (1967), *The child mental status examination,* New York: Basic Books.

Greenhill, L., Rieder, R., Wender, P., Buchsbaum, M., and Zahn, T. (1973), Lithium carbonate in the treatment of hyperactive children. *Arch. Gen. Psychiat., 28,* 636–640.

Hartlage, L. (1965), Effects of chlorpromazine on learning. *Psychological Bull., 64,* 235–45.

Hayes, T. A., Panitch, M. L., and Barker, E. (1975), Imipramine dosage in children: A comment on imipramine and electrocardiographic abnormalities in hyperactive children. *Am. J. Psychiat., 132,* 546–547.

Haywood, H. (1966), Perceptual handicap: Fact or artifact? *Child Study,* 1966, *28,* 2.

Huessy, H., and Wright, A. (1970), The use of imipramine in children's behavior disorders. *Acta Paedopsychiat., 37,* 194–99.

Ingram, R. (1956), A characteristic form of overactive behavior in brain damaged children. *J. Ment. Sci., 102,* 550–58.

Katz, S., Saraf, K., Gittelman-Klein, R., and Klein, D. (1975), Clinical pharmacological management of hyperkinetic children. *Int. J. Ment. Health, 4,* 157–181.

Kehne, C. (1974), *Social control of the hyperactive child via medication: At what cost to personality development: Some psychological implications and clinical interventions.* Presented at annual meeting, Orthopsychiatric Association.

Killam, E. (1968), Pharmacology of the reticular formation. In D. H. Efron (Ed.), *Psychopharmacology, A review of progress, 1957–1967.* Washington, D.C.: Public Health Service Publication No. 1836, pp. 411–445.

Klein, D., and Gittelman-Klein, R. (1975), Problems in the diagnosis of minimal brain dysfunction and the hyperkinetic syndrome. *Int. J. Ment. Health, 4,* 45–60.

Knights, R. and Hinton, G. (1969), The effects of methylphenidate (Ritalin) on the motor skills and behavior of children with learning problems. *J. Nerv. Ment. Dis., 148,* 643–653.

Knobel, M. (1962), Psychopharmacology for the hyperkinetic child: dynamic considerations. *Arch. Gen. Psychiat., 6,* 198–202.

Kraft, I. (1968), The use of psychoactive drugs in the outpatient treatment of psychiatric disorders of children. *Am. J. Psychiat., 124,* 1401–07.

Kupietz, S., Bialer, I., and Winsberg, B. G. (1972), A behavior rating scale for assessing improvement in behaviorally deviant children: A preliminary investigation. *Am. J. Psychiat., 128,* 1432–1436.

Laufer, M., Denhoff, E., and Solomons, G. (1957), Hyperkinetic impulse disorder in children's behavior problems. *Psychosom. Med., 19,* 38–49.

LeVann, J. L. (1971), Clinical comparison of haloperidol with chlorpromazine in mentally retarded children. *Am. J. Ment. Def., 75,* 719–723.

Levitt, E. (1957), The results of psychotherapy with children: An evaluation. *J. Consult. Psych., 21,* 189–96.

Levitt, E. (1963), Psychotherapy with children: A further evaluation. *Behavior Res. & Ther., 1,* 45–51.

McCarthy, J. (1973), Education: The base of the triangle. *Ann. N.Y. Acad. Sci., 205,* 362–367.

Mendelson, W., Johnson, N., and Stewart, M. A. (1971), Hyperactive children as teenagers: A follow-up study. *J. Nerv. Ment. Dis., 153,* 273–279.

Miller, N., and Cantwell, D. (1975), *Siblings as therapists: A behavioral approach.* Presented at the American Psychiatric Association meeting, Anaheim, Ca., May, 1975.

Millichap, J. (1973), Drugs in management of minimal brain dysfunction. *Ann. N.Y. Acad. Sci., 205,* 321–34.

Millichap, J. G., and Boldrey, E. (1967), Studies in hyperkinetic behavior: II. Laboratory and clinical evaluations of drug treatment. *Neurology, 17,* 467–471, 519.

Millichap, J., and Fowler, G. (1967), Treatment of 'mimimal brain dysfunction' syndromes. *Ped. Clin. N. Am., 14,* 767–777.

Millichap, J. G., Aymat, F., Sturgis, L. H., Larsen, K. W., and Egan, R. A. (1968), Hyperkinetic behavior and learning disorders: III. Battery of neuropsychological tests in controlled trial of methylphenidate. *Am. J. Dis. Ch.*, *116*, 232–244.

Minde, K., Lewin, D., Weiss, G., Lavigueur, H., Douglas, V., and Sykes, E. (1971), The hyperactive child in elementary school: A 5 year, controlled followup. *Exceptional Children*, *38*, 215–21.

Minde, K., Weiss, G., and Mendelson, M. (1972), A five-year follow-up study of 91 hyperactive school children. *J. Am. Acad. Ch. Psychiat.*, *11*, 595–610.

Montagu, J. D. (1975), The hyperkinetic child: A behavioural, electrodermal and EEG investigation. *Dev. Med. & Ch. Neurol.*, *17*, 299–305.

Morrison, J. R., and Stewart, M. A. (1971), A family study of the hyperactive child syndrome. *Biol. Psychiat.*, *3*, 189–195.

O'Malley, J. E., and Eisenberg, L. (1973), The hyperkinetic syndrome. *Sem. in Psychiat.*, *5*, 95–103.

Ounsted, C. (1955), The hyperkinetic syndrome in epileptic children. *Lancet*, *269*, 303–11.

Page, J. G., Bernstein, J. E., Janicki, R. S., and Michelli, F. A. (1972), *A multi-clinic trial of pemoline in childhood hyperkinesis*. Presented at the Symposium on the Clinical Use of Stimulant Drugs in Children, Key Biscayne, Fla.

Patterson, G. (1971), Behavioral intervention procedures in the classroom and in the home. In A. E. Bergin, and S. L. Garfield (Eds.), *Handbook of psychotherapy and behavior change*. New York: John Wiley and Sons, pp. 751–777.

Patterson, G., Jones, R., Whittier, J., and Wright, M. (1965), A behaviour modification technique for the hyperactive child. *Behaviour Res. and Ther.*, *2*, 217–26.

Peters, J., Davis, J., Goolsby, C., Clements, S., and Hicks, T. (1973), *Physician's handbook— screening for MBD*. CIBA Medical Horizons.

Pincus, J., and Glaser, G. (1966), The syndrome of 'minimal brain damage' in childhood. *New Eng. J. Med.*, *275*, 27–35.

Polizos, P., Engelhardt, D. M., and Hoffman, S. P. (1973), CNS consequences of psychotropic drug withdrawal in schizophrenic children. *Psychopharm. Bull.*, *9*, 34–35.

Pond, D. (1961), Psychiatric aspects of epileptic and brain-damaged children. *Brit. Med. J.*, *2*, 1377–82, 1454–59.

Psychopharmacology Bulletin (1973), Special Issue, Pharmacotherapy of children. NIMH, DHEW Publication No. (HSM) 73-9002.

Quinn, P., and Rapoport, J. (1975), One-year follow-up of hyperactive boys treated with imipramine or methylphenidate. *Am. J. Psychiat.*, *132*, 241–245.

Rachman, S. (1971), *The effects of psychotherapy*. Oxford: Pergamon Press.

Rapoport, J., Lott, I., Alexander, D., and Abramson, A. (1970), Urinary noradrenaline and playroom behaviour in hyperactive boys. *Lancet 2*, 1141.

Rapoport, J., Quinn, P., Bradbard, G., Riddle, K., and Brooks, E. (1974), Imipramine and methylphenidate treatments of hyperactive boys. *Arch. Gen. Psychiat.*, *30*, 789–793.

Rutter, M. (1968), Lésion cérébrale organique, hyperkinesie et retard mental. *Psychiatrie de l'enfant*, *11*, 475–492.

Rutter, M., Levbovici, S., Eisenberg, L., Sneznevskij, A., Sadoun, R., Brooke, E., and Lin, T. (1969), A tri-axial classification of mental disorders in childhood. *J. Ch. Psych. & Psychiat.*, *10*, 41–61.

Rutter, M., Graham, P., and Yule, W. (1970a), *A neuropsychiatric study in childhood*. Philadelphia: J. B. Lippincott Co.

Rutter, M., Tizard, J., and Whitmore, K. (1970b), *Education, health and behaviour: Psychological and medical study of childhood development*. New York: John Wiley and Sons.

Rutter, M., Shaffer, D., and Shepherd, M. (1974), An evaluation of the proposal for a multi-axial classification of child psychiatric disorders (the British study). Report to World Health Organization. To be published.

Safer, D., Allen, R., and Barr, E. (1972), Depression of growth in hyperactive children on stimulant drugs. *New Eng. J. Med.*, *287*, 217–20.

Safer, D., and Allen, R. (1973), Factors influencing the suppressant effects of two stimulant drugs on the growth of hyperactive children. *Pediatrics*, *51*, 660.

Satterfield, J. (1973a), Personal communication.

Satterfield, J. (1973b), EEG issues in children with minimal brain dysfunction. *Sem. in Psychiat.*, *5*, 35–46.

Satterfield, J., Cantwell, D. P., Saul, R. E., Lesser, L. I., and Podosin, R. L. (1973), Response to stimulant drug treatment in hyperactive children: Prediction from EEG and neurological findings. *J. Aut. & Ch. Schiz., 3,* 36–48.

Satterfield, J., Cantwell, D., and Satterfield, B. (1974), Pathophysiology of the hyperactive child syndrome. *Arch. Gen. Psychiat., 31,* 839–844.

Schain, R., and Reynard, C. (1975), Observations on effects of a central stimulant drug (methylphenidate) in children with hyperactive behavior. *Pediatrics, 55,* 709–716.

Schildkraut, J. J., and Kety, S. S. (1967), Biogenic amines and emotion. *Science, 156,* 21–30.

Schnackenberg, R. C. (1973), Caffeine as a substitute for Schedule II stimulants in hyperkinetic children. *Am. J. Psychiat., 130,* 796–798.

Shetty, J. (1971), Alpha rhythms in the hyperkinetic child. *Nature, 234,* 476.

Silver, Larry B. (1975), Acceptable and controversial approaches to treating the child with learning disabilities. *Pediatrics, 55,* 406–415.

Sprague, R. (1972), Psychopharmacology and learning disabilities. *J. Oper. Psychiat., 3,* 56–67.

Sprague, R. (1973), Minimal brain dysfunction from a behavioral viewpoint. *Ann. N.Y. Acad. Sci., 205,* 349–61.

Sprague, R., and Werry, J. (1971), Methodology of psychopharmacological studies with the retarded. In N. Ellis (Ed.), *International review of research in mental retardation,* Vol. V. New York: Academic Press, pp. 147–219.

Sprague, R., and Sleator, E. (1973), Effects of psychopharmacologic agents on learning disorders. *Ped. Clin. N. Am., 20,* 719–35.

Sprague, R., Christensen, D., and Werry, J. (1974), Experimental psychology and stimulant drugs. In C. K. Conners (Ed.), *Clinical use of stimulant drugs in children.* The Hague: Excerpta Medica, pp. 141–164.

Sprague, R., and Werry, J. (1974), Psychotropic drugs and handicapped children. In L. Mann, and D. Sabatino (Eds.), *Second review of special education.* Philadelphia: JSE Press, pp. 1–50.

Steinberg, G. S., Troshinsky, C., and Steinberg, H. C. (1971), Dextroamphetamine-responsive behavior disorder in children. *Am. J. Psychiat., 128,* 174–179.

Stewart, M., Pitts, F., Craig, A., and Dieruf, W. (1966), The hyperactive child syndrome. *Am. J. Orthopsychiat., 36,* 861–867.

Strauss, A., and Lehtinen, L. (1947), *Psychopathology and education of the brain-injured child.* New York: Grune and Stratton.

Tarjan, G., and Eisenberg, L. (1972), Some thoughts on the classification of mental retardation in the United States of America. *Am. J. Psychiat., Suppl.* 14–18, May 1972.

Waizer, J., Hoffman, S. P., Polizos, P., and Engelhardt, D. M. (1974), Outpatient treatment of hyperactive school children with imipramine. *Am. J. Psychiat., 131,* 587–91.

Ward, M. (1966), *Experimental modification of "hyperactive" behavior.* Unpublished B.S. thesis, Univ. of Ill.

Weiss, G., Werry, J., Minde, K., Douglas, V., and Sykes, D. (1968), Studies on the hyperactive child: V. The effects of dextroamphetamine and chlorpromazine on behavior and intellectual functioning. *J. Ch. Psych. and Psychiat., 9,* 145–156.

Weiss, G., Minde, K., Werry, J. S., Douglas, V. I., and Nemeth, E. (1971a), Studies on the hyperactive child: VIII. Five year follow-up. *Arch. Gen. Psychiat., 24,* 409–414.

Weiss, G., Minde, K., Douglas, V., Werry, J., and Sykes, D. (1971b), Comparison of the effects of chlorpromazine, dextroamphetamine and methylphenidate on the behavior and intellectual functioning. *Canad. Med. J., 104,* 20–25.

Weiss, G., Kruger, E., Danielsen, U., and Elman, M. (1975), Effect of long-term treatment of hyperactive children with methylphenidate. *Canad. Med. Ass. J., 112,* 159–165.

Wender, P. H. (1969), Platelet serotonin level in children with 'Minimal Brain Dysfunction,' *Lancet, 2,* 1012.

Wender, P. H. (1971), *Minimal brain dysfunction in children.* New York: Wiley-Interscience.

Wender, P. H. (1975), Speculations concerning a possible biochemical basis of minimal brain dysfunction. *Int. J. Ment. Health, 4,* 11–28.

Wender, P., Epstein, R., Kopin, I., and Gordon, E. (1971), Urinary monoamine metabolites in children with minimal brain dysfunction. *Am. J. Psychiat., 127,* 1411–1415.

Werry, J. S. (1972), Organic factors in childhood psychopathology. In H. Quay, and J. Werry (Eds.), *Psychopathological disorders of childhood.* New York: John Wiley and Sons, pp. 83–121.

Werry, J. S., Weiss, G., Douglas, V., and Martin, J. (1966), Studies on the hyperactive child: III. The effect of chlorpromazine upon behavior and learning ability. *J. Am. Acad. Ch. Psychiat.*, *5*, 292–312.

Werry, J. S., and Sprague, R. L. (1970), Hyperactivity. In C. G. Costello (Ed.), *Symptoms of psychopathology*. New York: John Wiley and Sons, pp. 397.

Werry, J. S., Sprague, R. L., Weiss, G., and Minde, K. (1970), Some clinical and laboratory studies of psychotropic drugs in children: An overview. In W. L. Smith (Ed.), *Drugs and cerebral function*. Springfield: Charles C. Thomas, pp. 134–144.

Werry, J., Minde, K., Guzman, A., Weiss, G., Dogan, K., and Hoy, E. (1972), Studies on the hyperactive child: VII. Neurological status compared with neurotic and normal children. *Am. J. Orthopsychiat.*, *42*, 441–450.

Werry, J. S., and Sprague, R. (1972), Psychopharmacology. In J. Wortis (Ed.), *Mental retardation*. Vol. IV. New York: Grune and Stratton, pp. 63–79.

Whitehead, P. L., and Clark, L. D. (1970), Effect of lithium carbonate, placebo and thioridazine on hyperactive children. *Am. J. Psychiat.*, *127*, 824–825.

Winsberg, B., Bialer, I., Kupietz, S., and Tobias, J. (1972), Effects of imipramine and dextroamphetamine on behavior of neuropsychiatrically impaired children. *Am. J. Psychiat.*, *128*, 1425–31.

Winsberg, B. G., Press, M., Bialer, I., and Kupietz, S. (1974), Dextroamphetamine and methylphenidate in the treatment of hyperactive/aggressive children. *Pediatrics*, *53*, 236–41.

Winsberg, B. G., Goldstein, S., Yepes, L. E., and Perel, J. M. (1975), Imipramine and electrocardiographic abnormalities in hyperactive children. *Am. J. Psychiat.*, *132*, 542–545.

Winsberg, B. G., Yepes, L., and Bialer, I. (in press), Psychopharmacological management of children with hyperactive/aggressive/inattentive behavior disorders: A guide for the pediatrician. *Clin. Ped.*

Witt, P., Ellis, M., and Sprague, R., Methylphenidate and free range activity in hyperactive children. Unpublished paper written in support of NIMH grant No. MH189–9, Children's Research Center, Univ. of Ill., Urbana.

Wong, G. H., and Cock, R. Z. (1971), Long-term effect of haloperidol on severely emotionally disturbed children. *Australian and New Zealand J. Psychiat.*, *5*, 296–300.

Zrull, P., Patch, D., and Lehtinen, P. (1966), Hyperkinetic children who respond to d-amphetamine. Scientific proceedings summary, American Psychiatric Association, Atlantic City, N.J.

Chapter Seven

TREATMENT OF
DEPRESSIVE STATES

Alexander R. Lucas, M.D.

THE CONCEPT OF DEPRESSION IN CHILDHOOD

Symptoms of sadness and misery in childhood are not difficult to recognize, yet depression continues to be among the most poorly understood emotional phenomena of childhood. When overtly depressed mood is manifest, it is readily apparent to parents, teachers, and professionals, but it is often disregarded as transient or unimportant. Depression in children is still poorly understood because there is no general agreement about the phenomenology and nosology, nor have its biological concomitants been defined. Mood changes are frequent among children. These may be acute and transient mood swings, episodes of sadness and misery in reaction to a host of environmental events, and more profound or lasting depressive conditions. Shaw (1966) differentiated unhappiness from depression in children. He identified unhappiness as the major symptom in psychiatry, the very reason for psychiatry's being. Within a large constellation of symptoms, including anxiety, depression, apathy, withdrawal, anger, fear, panic, and jealousy, unhappiness is subsumed. It is all of these, yet none of them. It is the absence of happiness. The absence of joy, of pleasure, and of delight is the essence of unhappiness. Unhappiness in a child seems doubly tragic because happiness and fun are among the natural rights of childhood.

Depressive reactions to environmental circumstances are ubiquitous symptoms of childhood psychopatholody. Bowlby (1973) used as an inscription for his chapter on "Prototypes of Human Sorrow" a passage from Graham Greene's *A Sort of Life:* "Unhappiness in a child accumulates because he sees no end to the dark tunnel."

When events are viewed by the child as so overwhelming that there is no solution, depression occurs. In the young child security and assurance that all will be right come from the parents. Therefore, potentially harmful situations will not cause depression in the child if the parents continue to protect the child, and if the child maintains faith in the parents' omnipotence. If there is loss of a parent, the child is at risk to develop depression. When deprived of both parents for an extended period of time, depression is almost certain to occur.

Separation and loss are the common denominators in depressions of childhood. The loss may be real as in the death of a parent, or due to prolonged separation. It may be symbolic in relation to the emotional interaction between parent and child, as when a parent is psychotic or depressed and unable to provide the child with necessary affective interaction.

Hill (1968) classified depression in terms of reaction, posture, and disease. Graham (1974) commenting on this classification, expressed the opinion that to view childhood depression as a disease may be the least useful. This is consonant with the traditional view in child psychiatry that holds depression to be reactive. As such, intrapsychic and neurotic conflicts are implied. Those espousing this view tend to conceptualize the treatment in psychotherapeutic terms. Others, particularly European workers, have viewed childhood depressions as analogous to depressive illnesses of adulthood. These workers tend to rely more on biologic modes of treatment.

While there are some common threads which are discernible, depression takes on multiple appearances throughout the human life cycle (Cytryn and McKnew, 1974).

INFANCY AND YOUNG CHILDHOOD: PROTOTYPE OF DEPRESSION

The depressive position as a developmental phenomenon has been ascribed to young infants by some theorists such as Klein (1932). She attributed elaborate fantasies to the mental life of infants in terms of libidinal and aggressive wishes. The depressive position which she saw as the expression of a primary death instinct was viewed as the antecedent of later depressions (1948). The validity of these concepts has been questioned by others (Zetzel, 1953). Negative affect in infancy can be seen as a reaction to physiologic discomfort. Thus crying may not be dependent on intrapsychic conflicts, but an adaptive mechanism necessary for survival, as suggested by Graham (1974). It thus assumes important communicative value as one of the component instinctual responses upon which attachment to the mother is based (Bowlby, 1958).

Most modern writers tend to think of depressive symptoms as reactions to overwhelming loss. Studies of infants and young children who are separated from their mothers delineated clinical syndromes analogous to depressions of adulthood. The symptoms observed in these children resembled those of severe depressions in adults. Moreover, the symptoms were the result of the loss of the mother after a close tie to her had been established. Spitz called this condition anaclitic depression. Infants deprived of their mothers became weepy and demanding. They lost weight and failed to develop adequately. Subsequently they refused contact with others, developed insomnia, motor retardation, and became susceptible to diseases. If their mother was restored within three to five months, recovery occurred (Spitz and Wolf, 1946). A more grave condition, hospitalism, supervened if the mother was not restored. Total emotional deprivation for periods lasting longer than five months resulted in motor retardation, complete passivity, vacuousness, and decline in the developmental quotient (Spitz, 1945).

The observations of Robertson and Bowlby (1952) on children in institutions and hospitals separated from their mothers resembled those of Spitz. They led to the delineation of a sequence of responses termed protest, despair, and detachment. Bowlby (1951) described the infant's response to separation as a form of depression having many of the hallmarks of the typical adult depressive patient. He described the infant as listless, quiet, unhappy, and unresponsive to a smile or coo. The emotional tone was one of apprehension and sadness. There was withdrawal from the child's surroundings and cessation of contact with strangers. The child's activities were retarded resulting in inert posture or stupor. Lack of sleep and appetite led to loss of weight and susceptibility to infection. A sharp drop in general development occurred. The long-term consequences of prolonged deprivation of maternal care were evaluated by Bowlby in his study of the world literature. Far-reaching effects on the child's character resulted, leading to the "affectionless" personality and delinquent character.

CHILDHOOD

The above-mentioned symptoms are characteristic of the very young child in reaction to separation from his mother. As the child grows, a wider repertory of behaviors becomes possible in reaction to frustration and stress. In the second year the child characteristically responds by opposition (Levy, 1955). In the third and fourth years of life, a variety of behaviors is possible, yet the reactions of a particular child are strongly influenced by temperamental characteristics and are somewhat predictable (Chess et al., 1960).

Clinical Manifestations

Shaw and Lucas (1970a) described depression in school-age children as presenting a picture of sadness, disinterest, and general psychomotor diminution (slowing of activity, constriction of emotional responses, and slowed mentation). It results when the child, finding no escape from conflict or from overwhelming events in the environment, finally gives up the struggle. Before reaching the point of despair, the child may react in a variety of ways: through guilt, resignation, anxiety symptoms, somatic symptoms, restlessness, or rebellion. Overt depression supervenes after other attempts to cope with the situation—adaptive mechanisms or rebellious reaction—have failed. Often the child will be unable to verbalize feelings of depression. Yet the change in his behavior is ample signal that something is wrong.

From the standpoint of ego psychology, Bibring (1953) viewed depression as the emotional expression of a state of helplessness and powerlessness. He stressed the importance of loss of self-esteem, a symptom pervasively present in children who are depressed.

Using the Hampsted Diagnostic Profile as a guide, Sandler and Joffe (1965) enumerated the symptoms that many depressed children had in common:

1. sad, unhappy appearance
2. withdrawal, constriction of interest, appearance of boredom
3. discontent, not readily satisfied, little capacity for pleasure
4. communicating a sense of feeling rejected or unloved
5. not prepared to accept help or comfort
6. tendency to regress to passivity
7. insomnia
8. persistent autoerotic or other repetitive activities
9. difficulty in making sustained contact with therapist

Malmquist (1971) noted some additional signs and symptoms based on his experience in treating depressed children:

10. physical or vegetative signs—headaches or abdominal complaints, dizziness, sleeping or eating disturbances
11. low frustration tolerance and irritability coupled with self-punitive behavior
12. reversal of affect by clowning or foolish behavior
13. denial of feelings of helplessness and hopelessness
14. provocative behavior eliciting scapegoating
15. self-criticalness
16. obsessive-compulsive behavior
17. episodic acting-out behavior

Depression in children is often expressed by somatic symptoms. Abdominal pain, constipation, headache, vomiting, transient migratory aches and pains may reflect feelings of depression. When such symptoms recur frequently, when the symptoms do not fit a physical disease, and when a physical cause cannot be found, emotional conflicts in the child and family should be investigated. Glaser (1967) called attention to the occurrence of masked depressions in children and adolescents, pointing out that depression is often not recognized because it is hidden by behavioral symptoms and delinquent behavior such as temper tantrums, disobedience, truancy, and running away from home. Psychoneurotic reactions such as school phobia and failure to achieve in school can mask underlying depression, as can psychophysiologic reactions. Lesse (1974) also noted that a variety of acting-out patterns may mask depression in children. The study of clinical characteristics of overtly depressed children by Poznanski and Zrull (1970) revealed that most demonstrated aggressive symptomatology including violent explosive outbursts.

In an ongoing study of depression in latency-age children, Cytryn and McKnew (1972) identified three distinct categories based on clinical phenomenology:

1. masked depressive reactions
2. acute depressive reactions
3. chronic depressive reactions

Masked depressions characterized by hyperactivity, aggressive behavior, psychosomatic illness, hypochondriasis, and delinquency were the most frequent. Clinically, depression and severe self-denigration were discernible. Acute depressions manifested by withdrawal, depressed affect, sleep disturbance, lack of appetite, school failure, and separation anxiety followed a sudden loss. These children had a good premorbid adjustment and an absence of depression in the parents. Chronic depressive reactions were seen in children with marginal premorbid social adjustment, often with inadequate early life experiences and previous depressive episodes. They demonstrated severe depressed mood, insomnia, anorexia, weight loss, and the presence of depression in at least one parent (McKnew and Cytryn, 1973).

Vulnerability Factors

There are factors, both biologic and environmental, that sensitize the child to make him vulnerable to depression. They include genetic predisposition, physical and sensory handicaps, deprivation, separation, parental illness (physical and emotional), parental loss, other losses, physical illness, and hospitalization. Repeated losses increase the risk of vulnerability.

Endogenous Depressions of Childhood

There are rare reports of manic-depressive illness in childhood and adolescence. The consensus is that true manic-depressive psychosis is exceedingly rare before puberty and almost unknown in earlier childhood (O'Gorman, 1965). Anthony and Scott (1960) reviewed the concept of manic-depressive psychosis in childhood; Dahl (1972) presented a further report. There is no doubt that some children manifest marked mood swings which in Europe are termed cyclothymic temperament. Some writers believe that this temperament is a prelude to the development of manic-depressive psychosis in later life (O'Gorman, 1965). Those who hold this view tend to favor the use of antidepressant drugs and lithium as treatment. American workers are more apt to label similar behavior hyperkinesis and prescribe stimulants or treat the situation psychotherapeutically. These geographic and philosophic differences highlight the importance of a careful diagnostic evaluation of the child, his family, and his environmental situation.

ADOLESCENCE

In adolescence the picture of depression can resemble that in earlier childhood or take on the appearance of adult depression. Furthermore, the characteristic changeability and extreme mood swings of normal adolescence may make it particularly difficult to differentiate phase-appropriate behavior from the pathological. The degree and the perseverance of troublesome behavior should alert the physician to investigate a problem in depth (Lucas, 1966). Moreover, when the behavior is out of character or presents a severe personality change, such an investigation should always be made.

Endogenous depressions of the unipolar or bipolar type often begin in adolescence. The first episode may be mild and go undetected. The physician should be alert to the possibility of depression when vague physical complaints persist and when apathy and lethargy are more than transient complaints. Persistent depressed affect, sleep and appetite disturbances, withdrawal, and vegetative signs are signals of serious depressive illness. The alarming rate at which suicide among teenagers is increasing is ample reason for eliciting the symptoms of depression and for asking about suicidal ideation (Renshaw, 1973). Among adolescents and youth, suicide is now the second greatest cause of death (Cantor, 1975).

CLASSIFICATION OF DEPRESSIVE STATES
IN CHILDHOOD AND ADOLESCENCE

There is as yet no generally accepted classification of depressive states in childhood and adolescence. One approach to classification is to consider the age of the child. Cytryn and McKnew (1972) divided depressive reactions phenomenologically into the acute, the chronic, and the masked. A more complete but necessarily imperfect approach considers etiology as the basis for categorization. Malmquist (1971) suggested a classification combining the three criteria: age, phenomenology, and etiology. Ultimately a classification based on etiology will provide the soundest basis for treatment. Table 1 outlines a tentative scheme comparing the three approaches.

TABLE 1

Classification of Depressive States in Children and Adolescents

Age	Phenomenology (Cytryn and McKnew, 1972)	Etiology
1. Infancy	1. Masked depressive reaction	1. Deprivation states
2. Early childhood		a. anaclitic depression (Spitz and Wolf, 1946)
3. Mid-childhood	2. Acute depressive reaction	b. hospitalism (Spitz, 1945)
4. Adolescence		2. Depression associated with organic disease (Malmquist, 1971)
	3. Chronic depressive reaction	3. Reactive depressions
		a. to loss
		(1) actual
		(2) symbolic
		b. to separation
		c. to injury
		d. to physical illness
		e. to parental illness
		(1) physical
		(2) emotional
		f. to severely disorganized environment
		g. to impaired self-esteem
		4. Masked depressions (Glaser, 1967)
		5. Depressive illness (endogenous unipolar)
		6. Manic-depressive illness (endogenous bipolar)

The vast majority of depressions of childhood are reactive. This includes those conditions in reaction to gross deprivation and the masked depressions. Exceptions are the endogenous depressions and those depressions which are an integral part of an organic disease process. Endogenous depressions have already been considered. Reactive depression to physical illness should be distinguished from those depressions which are associated with a serious disease process itself. Children with the latter condition may have a more profound neurochemical change akin to the disturbances thought to occur in endogenous depressions. Langford (1961) noted what he termed "organismic anxiety" in children who unconsciously perceived a threat to their lives or the integrity of their bodies.

TREATMENT OF DEPRESSION

General Principles

The rational approach to the treatment of reactive depressions is the alleviation of those influences that have set the stage for the depression, and of those that perpetuate it. Careful diagnostic evaluation of the child and family will most often elucidate those influences. Appropriate intervention at the individual, family, school, and/or community levels is then the desired treatment. In the direct treatment of the child, attention to impaired self-esteem is of paramount importance. When the child's coping mechanisms are inadequate or when environmental influences are overwhelming, placement of the child in a neutral or therapeutic setting is indicated.

McKnew and Cytryn (1975) emphasized early detection of childhood depression and emphasized also the importance of detection and treatment of depressed parents and of chaotic family situations. The aims of therapy as formulated by McKnew and Cytryn are to decrease self-depreciation and sense of rejection. Increasing self-esteem and ego strength is stressed. Brief hospitalization in some cases was found to be an effective form of crisis intervention.

Psychopharmacologic Treatment

It is plausible to assume that changes in the biogenic amine metabolism underlying endogenous depressions of childhood and adolescence are analogous to those postulated to occur in adult affective disorders. It is even possible that changes in brain amines occur secondarily in reactive depressions. If these speculations are correct, it would be logical to treat the conditions with drugs capable of altering the metabolism of the biogenic amines (norephinephrine, dopamine, and serotonin) thereby restoring normal mood. Considerable knowledge exists about the biochemical substrate of mood disorders in adults, and there has been major progress in recent years in pharmacologic treatment. Unfortunately the situation is far from encouraging as it pertains to children. Virtually nothing is known about the biochemical changes associated with mood alterations in children. Moreover, little is understood about the pharmacodynamics and pharmacokinetics of psychoactive drugs in children. The rates of absorption and excretion, the maintenance of blood levels, individual differences in drug metabolism, and drug interactions all are as yet poorly understood. Alterations in biogenic amine metabolism as a function of development are only beginning to be studied.

There is, therefore, as yet no completely rational basis for the drug treatment of depressions in children. Some empirical data exist, but reports are for the most part anecdotal and difficult to evaluate objectively.

The role of drugs in the treatment of depressions of childhood is a limited one. Major reviews on psychopharmacology in childhood, when they make note of drug treatment of depression at all, give it only cursory attention (Freedman, 1958; Bender and Faretra, 1961; Eveloff, 1966, 1970; Lucas, 1966, 1971; Freeman 1966; Fish, 1967, 1968; Eisenberg, 1968; Shaw and Lucas, 1970a; Renshaw, 1975; Conners, 1975). Standard textbooks of psychopharmacology often omit mention of antidepressant drugs in children altogether. The reason is clear. Very few relevant studies have been done. Nonetheless, it is not unusual for child psychiatric practitioners to use antidepressant drugs with children and with adolescents. In practice they are used much more widely than the literature would suggest. While the greatest quantity of these drugs is undoubtedly prescribed for enuresis and for hyperactive behavior, the use of antidepressant drugs for depressed children is not uncommon in practice.

It is true that there is great diversity of opinion among physicians about the indications for antidepressant drugs and, in general, their use for depressive conditions in childhood finds marked differences on the two sides of the Atlantic. These divergent attitudes are epitomized by the following statements: "Inasmuch as depression, particularly in the form which is amenable to antidepressants, does not occur in children and but rarely in adolescents, the antidepressants which are so useful in the treatment of severe depressions in adults, have no real role to play in childhood psychopharmacology." (Werry, 1967.) "Evidence is accumulating that [depressive illness] forms a significant problem in child health. . . . The prognosis in the case of depressed children receiving antidepressive treatment is very good, but if untreated most continue to remain ill for years." (Frommer, 1968.)

In North America, treatment for childhood depressions has been chiefly through environmental manipulation and psychotherapy; antidepressant drugs are more widely employed by European child psychiatrists. There are exceptions among both geographic groups, yet there is general agreement that when used, drugs must be but *part* of the treatment program with attention paid to the whole child, his family, the school situation, and the larger environment.

CLASSIFICATION OF MOOD-ALTERING DRUGS

The pharmacologic classification of antidepressant drugs includes the central nervous system stimulants, the monoamine oxidase inhibitors, and the tricyclic (iminodibenzyl) derivatives (Table 2). In addition, another mood-altering drug, lithium, should be included in a separate category of pharmacologic agents.

TABLE 2
Mood-Altering Drugs

1. CENTRAL NERVOUS SYSTEM STIMULANTS
      amphetamine (Benzedrine)
      dextroamphetamine (Dexedrine)
      methamphetamine (Desoxyn)
      methylphenidate (Ritalin)
      pemoline (Cylert)
      deanol (Deaner)
2. MONOAMINE OXIDASE INHIBITOR ANTIDEPRESSANTS
    a. hydrazine derivatives
        iproniazid (Marsalid)
        phenelzine (Nardil)
        nialamide (Niamid)
        isocarboxazid (Marplan)
    b. nonhydrazine compounds
        tranylcypromine (Parnate)
        pargyline (Eutonyl)
3. TRICYCLIC (IMINODIBENZYL) DERIVATIVE ANTIDEPRESSANTS
      imipramine (Tofranil)
      desimipramine (Norpramin, Pertofrane)
      amitriptyline (Elavil)
      nortriptyline (Aventyl)
      protriptyline (Vivactil)
4. LITHIUM SALTS
      lithium carbonate (Eskalith, Lithane, Lithonate)

1. Central Nervous System Stimulants

The central nervous system stimulants, comprising chiefly amphetamine and amphetamine substitutes, have a euphoriant effect in adolescents and adults. They have been used for their short-term antidepressant effect in adults, but the phenomenon of rebound depression makes this use hazardous. The CNS stimulants are not indicated in the treatment of depression in children or adolescents. A discussion of their use in other childhood disorders will be found in chapters one, five, and nine.

2. Monoamine Oxidase Inhibitor Antidepressants

Iproniazid was the first of the MAO inhibitors to be used in psychiatry when it was found to be highly effective in the treatment of adult depressive disorders. Because of its hepatoxicity, it was ultimately withdrawn from the market. MAO inhibitors were first used in autistic children in an attempt to heighten their interest in the environment. Freedman (1958) administered iproniazid to autistic schizophrenic children. He found that they showed an increased awareness of their surroundings and some employed a greater use of language. Nialamide and phenelzine were used by Bender and Faretra (1961) for similar indications. Soblen and Saunders (1961) used phenelzine in a group of young patients with schizophrenia and behavior disorders. The MAO inhibitors were also tried in depressed adolescents and children. Bender and Faretra gave nialamide and phenelzine to depressed adolescents (1961). Connell (1965) recommended phenelzine for depressive reaction in adolescents in doses of up to 45 mg. daily. Frommer (1967) gave a combination of phenelzine and chlordiazepoxide to some depressed children and isocarboxazid to depressed children with functional somatic symptoms and behavior disorders. She preferred MAO inhibitor antidepressants for children with uncomplicated depressions manifested by irritability, weepiness, and a tendency to recurrent explosions of temper or misery. Children with a depressive phobic anxiety state who had typical depressive symptoms including weepiness, tension, explosiveness, and irritability were also found to respond best to drugs of the MAO inhibitor group. Frommer identified the latter group of depressed children as less moody and more apathetic with the following predominant symptoms: abdominal pain that led to frequent school absences, insomnia, anxiety, lack of confidence, and personality withdrawal. Usually, in treating this group, Frommer (1968) combined the antidepressant with a tranquilizer, chlordiazepoxide, by choice.

Severe side effects including hypertensive crises have occurred in some adult patients receiving these drugs. The possibility of dangerous blood pressure elevation following the concurrent administration of two MAO inhibitors or of a MAO inhibitor and a tricyclic antidepressant has precluded such combinations in the United States. In England, however, combinations have been prescribed. Sympathomimetic drugs, including amphetamines, and foods with high tyramine content (aged cheeses, certain alcoholic beverages, pickled herrings, and chicken livers) may also interact adversely with MAO inhibitors to precipitate hypertensive crises (Shaw and Lucas, 1970b).

3. Tricyclic (Iminodibenzyl) Derivative Antidepressants

This group which includes imipramine and its congeners differs chemically from the MAO inhibitors. The tricyclic structures of these drugs have greater similarity to the phenothiazine drugs. However, their primary pharmacologic action is an antidepressant one, substantiated in studies of adult depressed patients. These drugs require prolonged administration of from one to four weeks before the antidepressant effects are observed (Schildkraut, 1970). Some sedative properties, in addition to the antidepressant effect, have been noted. The major use of the tricyclic compounds in child psychiatry and pediatrics has been for alleviation of enuresis (MacLean, 1960; Alderton, 1965; Poussaint and Ditman, 1965; Martin, 1971). These drugs have potent anticholinergic effects as well as an influence on the level of sleep.

Bender and Faretra (1961) reported using imipramine in autistic children, who became more alert, made attempts to speak, and began to relate. Kurtis (1966) reported the use of nortriptyline with autistic children. Kraft et al. (1966) gave amitriptyline to children with behavioral disturbances. Krakowski (1965) used it for hyperkinesis and Rapoport (1965) also reported on the use of imipramine for this indication. There followed several reports on the use of imipramine as an antihyperkinetic agent in children (Huessey and Wright, 1969, 1970; Werry, 1967; Gross, 1973; Gittelman-Klein, 1974). Some have advocated imipramine for children with a variety of emotional disorders and for school-phobic children (McLaughlin, 1964; Rabiner and Klein, 1969; Gittelman-Klein and Klein, 1975).

Reports on the use of tricyclic drugs for their antidepressant effect in children are rare. Lucas et al. (1965) reported on a placebo controlled study of amitriptyline in a diagnostically heterogeneous group of children and adolescents ranging in age from ten to seventeen presenting with symptoms of depression. More than half, primarily the adolescents, showed improvement in some of the symptoms relating to their depression on daily dosages up to 75 mg. Foster (1967) treated a group of children ranging in age from three to eleven years, presenting with mixed symptomatology considered to be on the basis of psychoneurotic depression, with nortriptyline in dosages of 2–3.5 mg./kg. daily. Most of the children experienced symptomatic improvement within two to four weeks. Eichhorn (1960) treated young depressed patients with imipramine but was not impressed with the results. Connell (1965) recommended imipramine in doses up to 150 mg. per day in those depressions of adolescents similar to endogenous depressions of adulthood. McKnew and Cytryn (1975) noted that they were unimpressed with the results of tricyclic antidepressant drug treatment in children.

Perhaps the most outspoken advocate of antidepressant drug therapy in children has been Frommer (1967, 1968). She has recommended the use of imipramine, amitriptyline, and trimipramine (not available in U.S.A.) in a variety of depressive conditions of childhood. Amitriptyline was given by Frommer to children as young as two and one-half years at a dose of 2.5 mg. daily, and in dosages of up to 100 mg. per day for children above the age of ten. Imipramine was used for children aged eight to ten years in dosages ranging from 10 to 60 mg. per day and in correspondingly greater doses for older children. Trimipramine was used in doses ranging from 25 to 100 mg. per day in children and young adolescents ranging from eight years to fourteen years. Combined treatment with trimipramine and isocarboxazid (a MAO inhibitor) 10 to 20 mg. per day was used in children over the age of eight when there was a profound depression that did not respond to a single drug of the MAO inhibitor or tricyclic group, and in severe obsessions and rituals thought to be of a depressive nature. Frommer classified depressed children on the basis of their presenting symptomatology. For those depressed children with enuresis and/or encopresis whose predominant symptoms included moodiness, weepiness, and immaturity, she considered the drug treatment of first choice to be amitriptyline or an allied drug. Children with uncomplicated depression were treated with one of the MAO inhibitor drugs by choice, as were the third group of children, those with a depressive phobic anxiety state. Symptomatology of the children in these two groups is described above, in the section on MAO inhibitors. A fourth group was identified as neurotic, without depressive affect. They had a high incidence of physical problems, including developmental difficulties such as speech disorders, congenital abnormalities, and acute or serious chronic illness. Immaturity and marked detachment and apathy were predominant symptoms. Learning problems were frequent. These children were often subjected to parental deprivation. Abdominal pain, headache, nausea, and vomiting occurred also in this group, although not as conspicuously as with the depressive group. Drug treatment was not very helpful for children in the neurotic group in Frommer's experience. A fifth group of children who displayed depressive features with extreme forms of temper outbursts alternating with brief states of reasonableness, or continuous unconstructive activity out of keeping with environmental expectations, was described by Frommer. These were thought to have early manifestations of manic-depressive psychosis and were treated with lithium.

A recent double-blind study of depressed children treated with imipramine was reported by Weinberg et al. (1973). These children demonstrated a high incidence of hyperactivity, school phobia, enuresis, and other developmental behavior problems. The drug-treated children showed significantly more improvement in the resolution of the presenting problems than did nontreated depressed children or nondepressed children. This study came under criticism regarding the criteria for diagnosing depression, and for methodologic reasons (Drotar, 1974; Lerer and Lerer, 1974; Weinberg, 1974).

Simson (1975) advocates tricyclic depressants combined with psychotherapy for the treatment of depressed children and adolescents. He prefers amitriptyline for children, using doses up to 50 or 75 mg. daily. A latent period of several weeks is generally noted before antidepressant effect is evident. With adolescents fourteen years or older, Simson prefers imipramine in doses of up to 75 mg. per day. In those latency-age children who have rapid onset of depression with hopelessness and poor self-concept interfering with school performance, a combination of methylphenidate in the morning and amitriptyline in the evening is used. Simson observes that a more rapid antidepressant result is obtained with this combination. In depressed children with explosive irritability, phenothiazine medication, such as thioridazine, is added to the antidepressant.

The cumulative clinical experience indicates that when used cautiously in moderate doses, serious side effects do not occur. However, the drugs are potentially cardiotoxic. When inappropriately large doses are prescribed and when the drugs are accidentally ingested, serious side effects and deaths can occur (Goel and Shanks, 1974; Steel et al., 1967).

4. Lithium Salts

Lithium carbonate has come to occupy an important place in the treatment of hypomania and mania (Schildkraut, 1970). Since the initial report of Cade (1949) it has become recognized as the most specific psychiatric treatment. The predominant use, by far, has been in adults. The diagnosis of mania or hypomania in children is considerably controversial, not generally accepted, and very rarely made or reported. Clinical criteria for the diagnosis of manic or manic-depressive illness in childhood have not been defined or established.

A few trials of lithium in children and adolescents have been reported. Van Krevelen and Van Voorst (1959) reported on the case of a fourteen-year-old retarded boy who had a cyclic psychosis with alternating manic and depressive phases. The diagnosis remained unclear but he responded and sustained a favorable result with lithium treatment. Frommer (1968) mentioned the use of lithium for "hypomanic" children. Some improved on lithium alone, and other "hypomanic" children were treated in addition with antidepressant drugs. Dosages in children from five to fourteen years of age ranged from 50 to 250 mg. daily. Some children became depressed on lithium. Frommer stated that unless there are truly endogenous and disruptive mood swings, the depression in children is almost certainly made worse by lithium salts.

Annell (1969a, 1969b) reported on lithium in the treatment of children and adolescents with a wide variety of behavioral symptoms including typical mania and cyclic mood swings. Dyson and Barcai (1970) noted a favorable response to lithium in two children of lithium-responding parents. These two boys, aged eight and thirteen years, did not manifest typical mood swings of manic-depressive illness but presented with short attention span, low frustration tolerance, explosive anger, sulkiness, and depression. A controlled study comparing lithium and chlorpromazine treatment of ten severely disturbed children, aged three to six years, by Campbell et al. (1972) revealed greater diminution of symptoms with chlorpromazine than with lithium. The exception was a six-year-old boy with hyperactivity, explosive affect, and autoaggressiveness who improved markedly on lithium. He was grossly schizophrenic and had been unresponsive to antipsychotic drugs. His excitement, impulsivity, hyperactivity, and violent self-mutilating behavior improved greatly but his psychotic symptoms did not. Greenhill et al. (1973) administered lithium to nine severely hyperactive children ranging in age from seven to fourteen years who were unresponsive to drugs and psychotherapy. Lithium was compared to dextroamphetamine and placebo. Six children showed no improvement or a worsening of symptoms but two with affective symptoms improved transiently. Those who showed marked improvement with lithium had affective components to their disorders with lability, euphoria, and depression.

The reports of lithium administration to children show marked variability and individual differences in response. Children who showed a constellation of symptoms including affective excitement, explosiveness, impulsiveness, aggressiveness, and hyperactivity were the ones to respond. Daily doses of lithium ranged from 50 mg. in five-year-old children to 1,800 mg. in adolescents. Serum lithium levels can be measured, and patients receiving this treatment should be monitored routinely. In adults serum levels ranging from 0.5 mEq/l to 1.5 mEq/l. have been considered therapeutic. Levels within this range were usual when they were reported in the children's studies. Lithium does not have FDA approval for children under twelve years.

PRINCIPLES OF DRUG TREATMENT

Insufficient information is available about the psychopharmacologic treatment of depressive states in children to make specific recommendations about the indications for particular drugs, about dosages, and about their use in certain types of depression. The tricyclic drugs are more widely used than drugs of the MAO inhibitor group. Medications are more likely to be used in children when depressive symptomatology is severe or when there has been failure to respond to other methods of treatment. It must be remembered that antidepressant drugs are not approved by the FDA for use in children under the age of twelve years except for certain indications such as enuresis.

There is agreement among those who advocate pharmacotherapy for childhood depressions that sound principles of psychotherapy, family therapy, and attention to learning difficulties must be included in treatment planning.

Antidepressants are clearly indicated in severe depressions of adolescence, particularly in late adolescence, the more so when clinical features point to an endogenous depressive illness. For children older than twelve dosages comparable to those used in adult psychopharmacologic practice are usually needed.

There is evidence that lithium carbonate is effective in certain cases of manic excitement regardless of age but there is insufficient comparative data with phenothiazine or butyrophenone drugs to single out one drug as preferable.

CONCLUSIONS

The important principle in treating depressed children (as in the treatment of other psychiatric problems of childhood) is that treatment must be holistic. The child, family, school, and community situation should all be considered in the treatment planning.

The state of the art is such that, except for the indication in adolescent depressions, little in the way of specific recommendations about antidepressive medications can be made. *There is, in fact, no consensus about whether antidepressant drugs should be used at all in children.* If antidepressant drugs are used as a part of a total treatment plan, it is incumbent upon the physician to become thoroughly familiar with the particular drugs, to review the risk of side effects and overdose with parents of the child, to use discretion in dosage, and to provide adequate follow-up supervision for the child receiving medication.

The vast majority of depressions in childhood are reactive, and the treatment must be addressed to alleviation of the precipitating and perpetuating circumstances, both internal and external.

Severe reactive depressions and those inferred to be endogenous may be indications for adjunctive antidepressive drug therapy. The tricyclic antidepressants are preferred to the MAO inhibitors. Dosage levels are still empirical in the absence of pharmacokinetic data. Imipramine in doses of 10 to 60 mg./day for younger children and 75 to 150 mg./day in older children and adolescents has been recommended (Frommer 1967, 1968; Simson, 1975). Above 75 mg./day the dosage should be divided to avoid the potential for serious side effects (Goel and Shanks, 1974).

Critical reading of papers written by those who have the most experience with drugs reveals that the appropriate use of drugs requires sensitivity to the art of medicine. More studies are needed to compare drugs, to determine whether the addition of drugs to the usual techniques of treatment is superior to the usual techniques alone, and if superior, whether the advantages outweigh the risks. Our understanding will be greatly enhanced when studies include the measurement of drug levels in the blood, and when drug metabolism in children is better understood. There are known side effects and acute toxic effects of the drugs, but little is known about the possible long-term effects in children. Conservatism in prescribing drugs for children is the paramount rule. Drugs should be used only when definite benefits will be derived that cannot be achieved by other means, and when the benefits are likely to outweigh the risks. Indiscriminate prescribing, the wholesale application of drugs to children with particular symptom clusters, the use of excessive doses, and the use of drugs as the sole treatment modality, are practices to be abhorred. Informed use of selective psychopharmacotherapy as an integrated part of the treatment program, on the other hand, is sound practice of medicine.

References

Alderton, H. R. (1965), Imipramine in the treatment of nocturnal enuresis of childhood. *Canad. Psychiat. Assn. J.*, *10*, 141–151.

Annell, A-L (1969a), Lithium in the treatment of children and adolescents. *Acta Psychiatrica Scand.*, (Suppl.), *207*, 19–33.

Annell, A-L (1969b), Manic-depressive illness in children and effect of treatment with lithium carbonate. *Acta paedopsych.*, *36*, 292–301.

Anthony, J., and Scott, P. (1960), Manic-depressive psychosis in childhood. *J. Ch. Psych. & Psychiat.*, *1*, 53–72.

Bender, L., and Faretra, G. (1961), Organic therapy in pediatric psychiatry. *Dis. Nerv. Sys.*, (Suppl. 4), *22*, 110–11.

Bibring, E. (1953), The mechanism of depression. In P. Greenacre (Ed.), *Affective disorders*. New York: Int. Univ. Press, pp. 13–48.

Bowlby, J. (1951), *Maternal care and mental health*. Geneva: WHO.

Bowlby, J. (1958), The nature of the child's tie to his mother. *Int. J. of Psycho-Anal.*, *39*, 350–373.

Bowlby, J. (1973), Attachment and loss, Vol. II: Separation. New York: Basic Books.

Cade, J. F. J. (1949), Lithium salts in the treatment of psychotic excitement. *Med. J. Austr.*, *2*, 349–352.

Campbell, M., Fish, B., Korein, J., Shapiro, T., Collins, P., and Koh, C. (1972), Lithium and chlorpromazine: a controlled crossover study of hyperactive severely disturbed young children. *J. Aut. & Ch. Schiz.*, *2*, 234–263.

Cantor, P. (1975), The effects of youthful suicide on the family. *Psychiatr. Opin.*, *12*, 6–11.

Chess, S., Thomas, A., Birch, H., and Hertzig, M. (1960), Implications for a longitudinal study of child development for child psychiatry. *Am. J. Psychiat.*, *117*, 434–441.

Connell, P. H. (1965), Suicidal attempts in childhood and adolescence. In J. G. Howells (Ed.), *Modern perspectives in child psychiatry*. Springfield: Charles C. Thomas, pp. 403–427.

Conners, C. K. (1975), Child psychiatry: organic therapies. In A. M. Freedman, H. I. Kaplan, and
   B. J. Sadock (Eds.), *Comprehensive textbook of psychiatry* Vol. II, 2nd Ed. Baltimore: Williams
   and Wilkins, pp. 2240–2246.
Cytryn, L., and McKnew, D. H., Jr. (1972), Proposed classification of childhood depression. *Am. J.
   Psychiat., 129,* 149–155.
Cytryn, L., and McKnew, D. H., Jr. (1974), Factors influencing the changing clinical expression of
   the depressive process in children. *Am. J. Psychiat., 131,* 879–881.
Dahl, V. (1972), A Follow-up study of child psychiatric clienteles with special regard to manic-
   depressive psychosis. In A-L. Annell (Ed.), *Depressive states in childhood and adolescence,*
   New York: Halstead.
Drotar, D. (1974), Concern over the categorization of depression in children (letter). *J. Ped., 85,*
   290–291.
Dyson, W. L., and Barcai, A. (1970), Treatment of children of lithium-responding parents. *Curr.
   Ther. Res., 12,* 286–290.
Eichhorn, O. (1960), Die Behandlung von Depressionen bei Jugendlichen. *Wien Medizin, Wo-
   chenschr., 110,* 747–748.
Eisenberg, L. (1968), Psychopharmacology in childhood: a critique. In E. Miller (Ed.), *Foundations
   of child psychiatry*. Oxford: Pergamon Press, pp. 625–641.
Eveloff, H. H. (1966), Psychopharmacologic agents in child psychiatry. *Arch. Gen. Psychiat., 14,*
   472–481.
Eveloff, H. H. (1970), Pediatric psychopharmacology. In W. G. Clark, and J. del Giudice (Eds.),
   Principles of psychopharmacology. New York: Academic Press, pp. 682–694.
Fish, B. (1967), Psychiatric treatment of children: organic therapies. In A. M. Freedman, and H. I.
   Kaplan (Eds.), *Comprehensive textbook of psychiatry,* Baltimore: Williams and Wilkins,
   pp. 1468–1472.
Fish, B. (1968), Drug use in psychiatric disorders of children. *Am. J. Psychiat., 124,* 31–36.
Foster, P. G. (1967), Treatment of childhood depression: use of nortriptyline (Aventyl). *Newton-
   Wellesley Med. Bull., 19,* 33–36.
Freedman, A. M. (1958), Drug therapy in behavior disorders. *Pediat. Clin. N. Am., 5,* 573–594.
Freedman, R. D. (1966), Drug effects on learning in children: A selective review of the past thirty
   years. *J. Spec. Ed., 1,* 17–44.
Frommer, E. A. (1967), Treatment of childhood depression with antidepressant drugs. *Brit. Med. J.,
   1,* 729–732.
Frommer, E. A. (1968), Depressive illness in childhood. In *Recent developments in affective disorders, Brit. J. Psychiat.,* Spec. Publ. No. 2, pp. 117–136.
Gittelman-Klein, R. (1974), Pilot clinical trial of imipramine in hyperkinetic children. In C. K. Conners (Ed.), *Clinical use of stimulant drugs in children,* Amsterdam: Excerpta Medica,
   pp. 192–201.
Gittelman-Klein, R., and Klein, D. F. (1975), School phobia: diagnostic considerations in the light
   of imipramine effects. In D. F. Klein, and R. Gittelman-Klein (Eds.), *Progress in psychiatric
   drug treatment*. New York: Brunner/Mazel, pp. 824–846.
Glaser, K. (1967), Masked depression in children and adolescents. *Am. J. Psychother., 21,*
   565–574.
Goel, K. M., and Shanks, R. A. (1974), Amitriptyline and imipramine poisoning in children. *Brit.
   Med. J., 1,* 261–263.
Graham, P. (1974), Depression in pre-pubertal children. *Dev. Med. Ch. Neurol., 16,* 340–349.
Gross, M. D. (1973), Imipramine in the treatment of minimal brain dysfunction in children. *Psycho-
   somatics, 14,* 283–285.
Greenhill, L. L., Rieder, R. O., Wender, P. H., Buchsbaum, M., and Zahn, T. P. (1973), Lithium
   carbonate in the treatment of hyperactive children. *Arch. Gen. Psychiat., 28,* 636–648.
Hill, D. (1968), Depression: disease, reaction, posture. *Am. J. Psychiat., 125,* 445–457.
Huessy, H. R., and Wright, A. L. (1969), Graded imipramine regimen favored in hyperkinetic
   children. *J.A.M.A., 208,* 1613–1614.
Huessy, H., and Wright, A. L. (1970), The use of imipramine in children's behavior disorders. *Acta
   Paedopsychiat., 37,* 194–199.
Klein, M. (1932), *The psycho-analysis of children*. London: Hogarth Press.
Klein, M. (1948), A contribution to the psychogenesis of manic-depressive states. In M. Klein, *Con-
   tributions to psycho-analysis*. London: Hogarth Press, pp. 282–310.

Kraft, I. A., Ardali, C., Duffy, J., Hart, J., and Pearce, P. R. (1966), Use of amitriptyline in childhood behavioral disturbances. *Int. J. Neuropsych., 2,* 611–614.

Krakowski, A. J. (1965), Amitriptyline in treatment of hyperkinetic children. *Psychosomatics, 6,* 355–360.

Kugel, R. B., and Alexander, T. (1963), The effect of a central nervous system stimulant (Deanol) on behavior. *Pediatrics, 31,* 651–655.

Kurtis, L. B. (1966), Clinical study of the response to nortriptyline on autistic children. *Int. J. Neuropsychiat., 2,* 298–301.

Langford, W. S. (1961), The child in the pediatric hospital: Adaptation to illness and hospitalization. *Am. J. Orthopsychiat., 31,* 667–684.

Lerer, R. J., and Lerer, M. P. B. (1974), Concern over the categorization of depression in children (letter). *J. Ped., 85,* 292.

Lesse, S. (1974), Depression masked by acting-out behavior patterns. *Am. J. Psychother., 28,* 352–361.

Levy, D. M. (1955), Oppositional syndromes and oppositional behavior. In P. H. Hoch, and J. Zubin (Eds.), *Psychopathology of childhood.* New York: Grune and Stratton.

Lucas, A. R. (1966), Psychopharmacologic treatment. In C. R. Shaw, *The psychiatric disorders of childhood.* New York: Appleton-Century-Crofts, pp. 387–402.

Lucas, A. R. (1971), Drug treatment for the troubled child. *Mich. Ment. Health Res. Bull., 5,* 5–22.

Lucas, A. R. (1975), Adolescence: phase or disturbance? *Minn. Med., 58,* 283–287.

Lucas, A. R., Lockett, H. J., and Grimm, F. (1965), Amitriptyline in childhood depressions. *Dis. Nerv. Syst., 26,* 105–110.

MacLean, R. E. G. (1960), Imipramine hydrochloride (Tofranil) and enuresis. *Am. J. Psychiat., 117,* 551.

Malmquist, C. P. (1971), Depressions in childhood and adolescence. *New Eng. J. Med., 284,* 887–893; 955–961.

Martin, G. I. (1971), Imipramine pamoate in the treatment of childhood enuresis. *Am. J. Dis. Ch., 122,* 42–47.

McKnew, D. H., and Cytryn, L. (1973), Historical background in children with affective disorders. *Am. J. Psychiat., 130,* 1278–1279.

McKnew, D. H., and Cytryn, L. (1975), Detection and treatment of childhood depression. Presented at Annual Meeting, American Psychiatric Assn., Anaheim, Ca., May 7.

McLaughlin, B. E. (1964), A double blind study involving thirty emotionally disturbed children (outpatients). *Psychosomatics, 5,* 40–43.

O'Gorman, G. (1965), The psychoses of childhood. In J. G. Howells (Ed.), *Modern perspectives in child psychiatry.* Springfield: Charles C. Thomas, pp. 472–495.

Poussaint, A. F., and Ditman, K. S. (1965), A controlled study of imipramine (Tofranil) in the treatment of childhood enuresis. *J. Ped., 67,* 283–290.

Poznanski, E., and Zrull, J. P. (1970), Childhood depression: clinical characteristics of overtly depressed children. *Arch. Gen. Psychiat., 23,* 8–15.

Rabiner, C. J., and Klein, D. F. (1969), Imipramine treatment of school phobia. *Comprehens. Psychiat., 10,* 387–390.

Rapoport, J. (1965), Childhood behavior and learning problems treated with imipramine. *Int. J. Neuropsychiat., 1,* 635–642.

Renshaw, D. C. (1973), Depression in the young, *J.A.M.W.A., 28,* 542–546.

Renshaw, D. C. (1975), Psychopharmacotherapy in children. In F. J. Ayd (Ed.), *Rational psychopharmacotherapy and the right to treatment.* Baltimore: Ayd Medical Communications, pp. 131–150.

Robertson, J., and Bowlby, J. (1952), Responses of young children to separation from their mothers. *Courr. Cent. Int. Enf., 2,* 131–142.

Sandler, J., and Joffe, W. G. (1965), Notes on childhood depression. *Int. J. Psycho-Anal., 46,* 88–96.

Schildkraut, J. J. (1970), *Neuropsychopharmacology and the affective disorders.* Boston: Little, Brown and Co.

Shaw, C. R. (1966), *The psychiatric disorders of childhood.* New York: Appleton-Century-Crofts.

Shaw, C. R., Lockett, H. J., Lucas, A. R., Lamontagne, C. H., and Grimm, F. (1963), Tranquilizer drugs in the treatment of emotionally disturbed children: Inpatients in a residential treatment center. *J. Am. Acad. Ch. Psychiat., 2,* 725–742.

Shaw, C. R., and Lucas, A. R. (1970a), *The psychiatric disorders of childhood,* 2nd Ed., ch. seven, Psychoneurosis. New York: Appleton-Century-Crofts, p. 146.

Shaw, C. R., and Lucas, A. R. (1970b), *The psychiatric disorders of childhood,* 2nd Ed., ch. twenty, Psychopharmacologic Treatment. New York: Appleton-Century-Crofts, pp. 436–456.

Simson, C. B. (1975), Personal communication.

Soblen, R., and Saunders, J. C. (1961), Monoamine oxidase inhibitor therapy in adolescent psychiatry. *Dis. Nerv. Sys., 2,* 96–100.

Spitz, R. A. (1945), Hospitalism. *Psychoan. Study Ch., 1,* 53–74.

Spitz, R. A., and Wolf, K. M. (1946), Anaclitic depression. *Psychoan. Study Ch., 2,* 313–342.

Steel, C. M., O'Duffy, J., and Brown, S. S. (1967), Clinical effects and treatment of imipramine and amitriptyline poisoning in children. *Brit. Med. J., 3,* 663–667.

Van Krevelen, D. A. and Van Voorst, J. A. (1959), Lithium in der Behandlung einer Psychose unklarer Genese bei einem Jugendlichen. *Acta Paedopsych., 26,* 148–152.

Weinberg, W. A. (1974), Reply (letter). *J. Ped., 85,* 292–293.

Weinberg, W. A., Rutman, J., Sullivan, L., Penick, E. C., and Dietz, S. G. (1973), Depression in children referred to an educational diagnostic center: Diagnosis and treatment. *J. Ped., 83,* 1065–1072.

Werry, J. S. (1967), The use of psycho-active drugs in children. *Ill. Med. J., 131,* 785–787, 827.

Winsberg, B. G., Bialer, I., Kupietz, S., and Tobias, J. (1972), Effects of imipramine and dextroamphetamine on behavior of neuropsychiatrically impaired children. *Am. J. Psychiat., 128,* 1425–1431.

Zetzel, E. R. (1953), The depressive position. In P. Greenacre (Ed.), *Affective disorders.* New York: Int. Univ. Press, pp. 84–116.

Chapter Eight

TREATMENT OF MILD
SYMPTOMATIC ANXIETY STATES

Joseph H. Patterson, M.D. & Albert W. Pruitt, M.D.

INTRODUCTION

Minor tranquilizers and sedatives should not be used in the treatment of the transient behavior problems of children unless there is also a substantial counseling effort. However, the practitioner may be consulted because of complaints related to such diverse disturbances as acute grief reactions, anxiety, fear, failure to fall asleep, night terrors, sleepwalking, colic, hypochondriasis, or antisocial and delinquent behavior. These syndromes or symptoms are sometimes amenable to treatment with minor tranquilizers, antihistamines, hypnotics, or anticonvulsants, and it is the purpose of this chapter to consider the appropriateness of such pharmacotherapy. Since minor emotional problems in childhood are often transient, the efficacy of drugs is difficult to establish. In fact there are few well-designed studies of minor tranquilizers, sedatives, and hypnotics in children.

With society's present emphasis on the avoidance of drug abuse, pediatricians may be reluctant to employ pharmacotherapy in school-aged children. In addition, the potential for accidental or intentional overdose must be considered. However, psychoactive drugs are used widely by practitioners who may not be aware of the presence of these agents in drug combinations used for many common disorders. Barbiturates, for example, are included in preparations for nausea (Emesert, WANS), asthma (Tedral, Quadrinal), and pain (Fiorinal, Daprisal).

Although counseling must be emphasized, psychotherapy also is not without danger (Eisenberg, 1971). The pediatrician must remember that sessions with the child and/or the parents, like the use of drugs, involve risks. If the practitioner is not trained to recognize and deal with the emotional and interpersonal conflicts, proper referral should be arranged.

As stated by Eisenberg and Conners (1971), psychoactive drugs in children "should be used only when a condition exists that requires treatment, when the agent prescribed is likely to be effective in treating that condition, when the likelihood of benefit outweighs the risk of toxicity and then only for the shortest period possible. Indeed, it is an error of equal magnitude to deny a patient an agent which can help relieve his symptoms and hasten his recovery." In prescribing psychoactive drugs for children as well as for patients of all ages the physician must not neglect his responsibility to establish the etiology and work toward a resolution of the behavior problems.

DISORDERS OF SLEEP

Sleep disorders include failure to fall asleep and disturbances during sleep. The complaints that most often come to the pediatrician are restless sleep, talking in sleep (somniloquy), nightmares, night terrors (pavor nocturnus), sleepwalking (somnambulism), irregular sleep habits, and difficulty getting to sleep. Restless sleep or repeated tossing while asleep usually only requires protection to keep the child from falling out of bed. Such activity while sleeping may accompany other types of sleep disturbance, such as somniloquy, which may disturb others in the household but usually does not arouse the child. In childhood, vocal sounds made during sleep are usually only broken words and sounds and probably accompany dreaming (Shirley and Kahn, 1958).

Nightmares and night terrors are sleep disruptions with different characteristics. The nightmare is a very vivid, terrifying dream that can be related in great detail at the time the child awakes, as well as the following morning. In contrast, when sleep is disturbed by a night terror the child, while not completely awake, appears in a state of panic and is difficult to console. He may appear disoriented and unfamiliar with the people and things about him. The following morning the child cannot recall the events.

Somnambulism may take place without the parents being aware that the child is out of bed. There is no evidence of fear and the child may seem confused or he may be able to perform rather complex tasks. When the episode is over, the child goes back to sleep and is unable to recall the event the following morning.

Stages of sleep are characterized by unique electroencephalographic patterns and classified as REM stage (rapid eye movement), stages one, two, three, and four. The child experiences each of these levels several times throughout the night, and some sleep disturbances occur primarily at a given level of sleep. For example, nightmares in children are associated with REM-stage sleep. Somnambulism occurs most often in the first third of the night and during stage four sleep. During the episode, the EEG pattern is persistently one of sleep rather than wakefulness. Night terrors may coexist with somnambulism or may occur alone. These events are also noted during stage four sleep. (Jacobson, Kales, and Kales, 1968). It has been suggested that drug therapy of severe sleep disturbances might be directed toward altering the level of sleep.

Drug Therapy of Sleep Disorders

Hypnotic drugs are among the oldest agents used by man. Chloral hydrate was first synthesized and used as a hypnotic in the mid-nineteenth century. It continues to be a very safe, useful drug for pediatric patients. The popularity of chloral hydrate decreased temporarily in the early twentieth century with the introduction of the barbituric acid derivatives. These compounds have had wide application in a number of conditions, including disorders of sleep. Many antihistamines also produce drowsiness and this side effect may be used to advantage in selected patients. Antihistamines and anticholinergic agents have been the primary ingredients in most nonprescription preparations to induce sleep.

A large number of other drugs have been manufactured for use as hypnotics. Newer benzodiazepines (flurazepam, Dalmane) are available for use in adult patients. Several compounds, such as ethchlorvynol (Placidyl), methaqualone (Quaalude), and glutethimide (Doriden), have not been approved for use in children by the Food and Drug Administration and should not be prescribed.

These agents are widely used in adult practice, but drug therapy is rarely necessary for sleep disturbances in children. Most pediatricians are aware of or have experienced the stimulated, excited child who was given a barbiturate at bedtime for sleep but reacted paradoxically. Barbiturates are sometimes used casually in treating restlessness and colic in infancy without absolute documentation of efficacy. One must remember other important effects of these agents, such as the induction of metabolic pathways that may lead to an increase in the rate of elimination of other exogenous or endogenous materials. For example, phenobarbital treatment was associated with a shortening of the plasma half-life of dexamethasone and an increase in dosage requirement of prednisone in patients with asthma (Brooks et al., 1972).

When a hypnotic agent is considered useful by the practitioner for a particular situation such as anxiety during hospitalization, loss of a family member, or other acute emotional stress, chloral hydrate (10–20 mg./kg. per day) or diphenhydramine (Benadryl, 1–2 mg./kg./day) may be used. Each of these agents has a large therapeutic index, a relatively short duration of action, and is available in convenient dosage forms.

However when chloral hydrate is used, its potential for drug interaction through competition of its metabolite (trichloroacetic acid) with other drugs for albumin binding sites must be remembered (Sellers and Koch-Weser, 1971). Clinically significant drug interactions have not been demonstrated for diphenhydramine, but if the antihistamine is used regularly, its efficacy as a hypnotic agent is likely to decrease (Teutsch et al., 1975).

After a careful investigation of the various factors that may influence sleep patterns, e.g., developmental stage, temperament, stress factors in environment, selected drugs may be prescribed for trial in some common disorders. In refractory and disturbing colic for which demonstrable organic causes are definitely excluded, phenobarbital elixir (up to 6 mg. diluted with water) may be used before each feeding for three to four days (Birdsong, 1975). The aim of this treatment is to interrupt the symptomatology that is so distressing to the mother and the infant. There also has been widespread use of atropine-barbiturate combinations (Donnatal, Sedadrops) for colic and restlessness; the usual dose is 0.25–0.50 cc. three or four times daily. However there are no well-designed studies to document efficacy.

The tricyclic antidepressant, imipramine, was reported effective in a small group of children with somnambulism and night terrors (Pesikoff and Davis, 1971), although no control group was included in that evaluation. The dose used was 10–50 mg. at bedtime, and there was complete cessation of the sleep disorder during the period of treatment. Additional clinical experience with similar dosages is needed before this drug can be recommended without qualification. Because the tricyclic antidepressants are extremely toxic in overdosage, this risk must be weighed against the potential benefit.

ANXIETY AND BEHAVIOR DISORDERS

Pharmacotherapy of anxiety, hyperactivity, and other disruptive or disturbing traits in children is difficult to categorize since diagnosis is frequently only a listing of symptomatology. The anxiety observed in children is often situational or developmental in origin, but in older children neurotic anxiety may develop. If drugs are to be used briefly to allay anxiety and fear, the physician also must be involved in correcting the distressing situation or seeking explanation for underlying conflicts. The first and essential procedure is a careful diagnostic evaluation.

When the physician is presented with complaints suggesting a psychological or developmental disturbance, e.g., disturbed or disturbing behavior, unusual fears or habit disorders, regressed or overly mature patterns, or symptoms of psychosomatic disorder, the following steps should be taken:

1. An interview with the parents, preferably both together, should be scheduled to obtain a detailed history of the presenting complaint(s), a developmental history including psychosocial as well as maturational milestones, and a sense of the family style and interactions.
2. A separate interview with the child to assess the mental status, establish a developmental level (including neurological status), and some direct gauge of the type and quality of the child's interpersonal relatedness. If the child is of older school age or adolescent, he or she may be seen initially with the parents or before the parents are interviewed.
3. In many cases, and whenever indicated by the nature of the difficulty, a report from the school is extremely helpful if not essential.
4. A determination may be made after steps one, two, or three that more specialized procedures such as psychological testing for intelligence, cognitive functioning and/or personality factors; tests for language and/or learning disabilities; or an EEG may be helpful for further diagnostic definition.
5. A determination can then be made of the nature of the disability:
   a. Acute or chronic.
   b. Primarily endogenous (e.g., learning disability, minimal brain dysfunction syndrome, developmental lag, mental retardation) or experiential.
   c. Developmental stress (transient phobic-like fears in the three- to five-year-old, sleep disturbance in the two-year-old).
   d. Reactive to inappropriate environmental pressures (for bowel and bladder control, for independence and self-sufficiency, for conformity or achievement) or to primary family disturbance.
   e. Internalized, persistent patterns of reaction, interaction and adaptation (e.g., relatively fixed symptoms, personality traits, character disorders, psychosomatic illness).
   f. More severe psychopathology, as in schizophrenic reactions, developmental deviations, or marked disruptions in essential functions.
6. A treatment plan is formulated on the basis of the above determinations. Management by the pediatrician or general physician may include medication, but only in combination with individual and/or family counseling. Drug therapy would more likely be advised when the problem is some combination of acute, reactive, or developmental stress, and/or a primarily endogenous disability, such as hyperactivity or minimal brain dysfunction. Complete reliance on medication without attention to the source or cause of the problem is ill advised. When the situation is of long standing, and is associated with identifiable environmental disturbance, or reflects internalized and fixed patterns, or is indicative of severe psychopathology, referral to a child psychiatrist or other specialized resource is indicated.

Sedatives and Minor Tranquilizers

Since sedative and hypnotic effects of drugs are difficult to separate, many of the agents used for sleep have also been used in lower dosage for control of anxiety. Drugs or groups of drugs which may be considered by the physician are: barbiturates, antihistamines, meprobamate, and benzodiazepines. These drugs have been used to control anxiety, but the pediatrician must always be reluctant to institute such drug therapy unless he is committed to supporting the child and the family in additional ways.

The barbiturates, especially phenobarbital, are the prototype against which the newer sedative agents have been compared. Although frequently forgotten, as mentioned earlier, barbiturates are added to medications for abdominal cramping and colic, asthma, aches and pain, nausea, and other disorders. The need for sedation in the treatment of such illnesses has not been proved.

During the Second World War a number of antihistamines were developed which were later shown to be histamine antagonist at the H_1 receptor (Beaven, 1976). In addition to their primary action, many of these compounds have a sedative, as well as an anticholinergic effect. Some drugs of this class that have sedative and hypnotic properties have been used in over-the-counter preparations for sleep. Diphenhydramine (Benadryl) was one of the earliest compounds synthesized in the systematic search for effective and safe antihistaminic agents. Because of its sedative properties, it has had some use in the treatment of behavior disturbances in young children.

Hydroxyzine (Atarax, Vistaril) was investigated in the early 1960s (Reagor, 1967–1968), and is an example of a chemical antihistamine with important sedative properties. In addition to oral and parenteral preparations of hydroxyzine, this compound is also included in a bronchodilator (Marax) and a gastrointestinal (Enarax) preparation. Just as in the case of the barbiturates, there is no proved justification for this combination.

Meprobamate and related drugs were developed in the search for longer-acting skeletal muscle relaxants. In clinical trials, the ataractic effect was noted and for several years this drug was widely used in adult practice.

Most recent developments of minor tranquilizers have been in the class of benzodiazepines. Chlordiazepoxide (Librium) was the first of these minor tranquilizers found to have significant antianxiety effect in the human (Randall and Schallek, 1968). Since the introduction of diazepam (Valium), several other benzodiazepines have been marketed for their sedative, hypnotic and anticonvulsant actions (Greenblatt and Shader, 1974a, 1974b). One theoretical advantage of meprobamate and the benzodiazepines over barbiturates is that the former agents do not appear to induce the microsomal enzyme systems in the liver that are responsible for the metabolism of a great many drugs and some endogenous compounds. However, the cost of these newer agents compared to the barbiturates must also be considered.

Although there are no well-controlled clinical studies of the use of benzodiazepines in emotional disorders of children, there are some pharmacokinetic data (Garattini et al., 1973). After oral administration, the peak blood level of diazepam occurs earlier in children than in adults and elderly subjects, but the plasma half-life of the drug is similar in these age groups.

A serious problem arises in the use of minor tranquilizers in the school-aged child since, as Irwin (1968) has pointed out, the sedative-hypnotics and minor tranquilizers in doses that are anxiolytic may impair cognitive functioning and coordination. In higher doses, drowsiness, ataxia, and muscle weakness occur. If undiagnosed depression is a prime factor in the patient's disturbance, the use of sedative agents may be detrimental.

Drug Therapy of Minor Behavior Disorders

There are few well-designed studies of sedative agents in outpatient children with minor behavior disorders. Most investigations of psychoactive agents in children have been carried out in institutionalized children with schizophrenia or other severe illness. Nevertheless there may be both chronic and acute situations (Kraft, 1968) called to the attention of the practicing pediatrician, in which a psychotropic agent is considered as adjunctive to a more definitive treatment program.

Some of the chronic behavior problems (Finch, 1958) about which the pediatrician may be consulted are: temper tantrums, rebellious behavior, sadistic and destructive behavior, impulsive and explosive outbursts. In addition to such aggressive types of behavior, the physician may also be faced with the child experiencing an acute psychological crisis (Lewis and Lewis, 1973) such as: the death of a sibling, death of a parent, or the impending death of the child. Acute and traumatic events in the environment may also temporarily affect the child's security and greatly increase his anxiety.

In earlier discussions of minor behavior problems in children (Finch, 1958; Lewis and Lewis, 1973), drug therapy was not considered seriously. In a monograph (Lewis and Lewis, 1973) devoted to the "Pediatric Management of Psychological Crises," the only psychoactive drug suggested was imipramine in the treatment of some children with school avoidance. Certainly this suggests "an unwarranted fear of psychopharmacological treatment, especially for nonpsychotic children and those with normal intellectual function" (Fish, 1968b). But drug therapy alone is not acceptable.

The antihistamine, diphenhydramine, has been evaluated in various behavior disorders of children (Effron and Freedman, 1953; Fish, 1960a, 1960b). The sedative properties of the drug were demonstrated, especially in children younger than ten years of age. Older children responded with drowsiness, rather than relief of anxiety, in much the same manner as adults. Even in these young children the aim was not complete relief of anxiety; instead it was to improve the child's ability to function and develop his own potential.

Meprobamate has also undergone trials in children with psychological disorders. In one study (Kraft et al., 1959) this drug reduced symptoms in several groups of disturbed children, when coupled with professional contact. In a group of nonpsychotic children (Cytryn et al., 1960), meprobamate, prochlorperazine and placebo were evaluated in conjunction with psychotherapy. The improvement in the two groups treated with the psychoactive agents was not statistically better than improvement in the placebo group. Since no group was followed without psychotherapy, it is not possible to know the incidence of spontaneous improvement in symptoms in these children.

The efficacy of the benzodiazepines in emotionally disturbed children has not had controlled study. Many investigations in adult patients (Greenblatt and Shader, 1974a, 1974b) have demonstrated the anxiolytic effect of several of these compounds, and the toxicity appears to be significantly less than that of the barbiturates. This is an important consideration in a family with young children, or in a severely depressed patient. However, the newer benzodiazepines are much more expensive than the older barbiturates.

Some investigators have considered anticonvulsants useful in the treatment of behavior disorders in children (Bender and Nichtern, 1956); these drugs, however, are generally effective only in patients with organic brain disease. A group of delinquent boys were treated with selected drugs, including diphenylhydantoin (Dilantin), without significant improvement in behavior (Conners et al., 1971).

CONCLUSION

In conclusion, there is no absolute documentation of benefit for the use of sedatives and minor tranquilizers in children. Clinical usage suggests that in uncommon situations, these drugs may be used briefly to advantage until the necessary counseling is achieved or until the acute situation has resolved. Of the drugs currently available, diphenhydramine, phenobarbital, and the benzodiazepines are most useful. Diphenhydramine appears to be poorly effective in behavior disorders of children older than ten years of age (Fish, 1968a); phenobarbital administration may result in a paradoxical hyperstimulated state; and the benzodiazepines are expensive.

Drugs are not a substitute for the care and caring that should be given by the health professional to the affected child and the parents.

References

Beaven, M. A. 1976, Histamine. *New Eng. J. Med. 294,* 320–325.

Bender, L., and Nichtern, S. 1956, Chemotherapy in child psychiatry. *N.Y. St. J. Med., 56,* 2791–2795.

Birdsong, Mc. 1975, Infantile Colic. In H. C. Shirkey (Ed.), *Pediatric therapy.* St. Louis: C. V. Mosby, pp. 617–617.

Brooks, S. M., Werk, E. E. Ackerman, S. J., Sullivan, I., and Thrasher, K. 1972, Adverse effects of phenobarbital on corticosteroid metabolism in patients with bronchial asthma. *New Eng. J. Med., 286,* 1125–1128.

Conners, C. K., Kramer, R., Rothschild, G. H., Schwartz, L., and Stone, A. 1971, Treatment of young delinquent boys with diphenylhydantoin sodium and methylphenidate. *Arch. Gen. Psychiat., 24,* 156–160.

Cytryn, L., Gilbert, A., and Eisenberg, L. 1960, The effectiveness of tranquilizing drugs plus supportive psychotherapy in treating behavior disorders of children: A double-blind study of eighty outpatients. *Am. J. Orthopsychiat., 30,* 113–129.

Effron, A. S., and Freedman, A. M. 1953, The treatment of behavior disorders in children with benadryl. *J. Ped., 42,* 261–266.

Eisenberg, L. 1971, Principles of drug therapy in child psychiatry with special reference to stimulant drugs. *Am. J. Orthopsychiat., 41,* 371–379.

Eisenberg, L., and Conners, C. K. 1971, Psycho-pharmacology in childhood. In N. B. Tabot, J. Kagan, and L. Eisenberg (Eds.), *Behavioral science in pediatric medicine.* Philadelphia: W. B. Saunders Co., pp. 397–423.

Finch, S. M. 1958, Office management of everyday problems. *Ped. Clin. N. Am., 5,* 561–572.

Fish, B. 1960a, Drug therapy in child psychiatry: Psychological aspects. *Compr. Psychiat., 1,* 55–61.

Fish, B. 1960b, Drug therapy in child psychiatry: Pharmacological aspects. *Compr. Psychiat., 1,* 212–227.

Fish, B. 1968a, Drug use in psychiatric disorders of children. *Am. J. Psychiat., 124,* 31–36, Suppl.

Fish, B. 1968b, Methodology in child psychopharmacology. In D. H. Effron (Ed.), *Psychopharmacology: A review of progress, 1957–1967.* Washington, D.C.: U.S. Public Health Service, Publ. No. 1836, pp. 989–1001.

Garattini, S., Marucci, F., Morselli, P. L., and Mussini, E. A. 1973, The significance of measuring blood levels of benzodiazepines. In D. S. Davies and B. N. C. Prichard (Eds.), *Biological effects of drugs in relation to their plasma concentration.* Baltimore: Univ. Park Press, 1973, pp. 211–225.

Greenblatt, D. J., and Shader, R. I. 1974a, Benzodiazepines. *New Eng. J. Med., 291,* 1011–1015.

Greenblatt, D. J., and Shader, R. I. 1974b, Benzodiazepines. *New Eng. J. Med., 291,* 1239–1243.

Irwin, S. 1968, Anti-neurotics: Practical pharmacology of the sedative hypnotics and minor tranquilizers. In D. H. Effron (Ed.), *Psychopharmacology: A Review of Progress, 1957–1967.* Washington, D. C.: U. S. Public Health Service, Publ. No. 1836, pp. 185–204.

Jacobson, A., Kales, J. D., and Kales, A. 1968, Clinical and electrophysiological correlation of sleep disorders in children. In A. Kales (Ed.), *Sleep physiology and pathology.* Philadelphia: J. B. Lippincott, pp. 109–118.

Kraft, I. A. 1968, The use of psychoactive drugs in the outpatient treatment of psychiatric disorders of children. *Am. J. Psychiat., 124,* 1401–1407.

Kraft, I. A., Marcus, I. W., Wilson, W., Swander, D. V., Rumage, N. S., and Schulhofer, E. 1959, Methodological problems in studying the effect of tranquilizers in children with specific references to meprobamate. *South. Med. J., 52,* 179–185.

Lewis, M., and Lewis, D. O. 1973, Pediatric management of psychologic crises. In S. Gellis, ed., *Current Problems in Pediatrics.* Chicago: Year Book Medical Publishers.

Pesikoff, R. B., and Davis, P. C. 1971, Treatment of pavor nocturnus and somnambulism in children. *Am. J. Psychiat., 129,* 134–137.

Randall, L. O., and Schallek, W. 1968, Pharmacological activity of certain benzodiazepines. In D. H. Effron (Ed.), *Psychopharmacology: A review of progress, 1957–1967.* Washington, D. C.: U. S. Public Health Service, Publ. No. 1836, pp. 153–184.

Reagor, P. A. 1967–1968, Five drugs used with children: A review of psychopharmacological research in the past decade. In R. L. Sprague, and J. S. Werry (Eds.), *Survey of research on psychopharmacology of children*. Urbana: Univ. of Ill. Press, pp. 248–268.

Sellers, E. M., and Koch-Weser, J. 1971, Kinetics and clinical importance of displacement of warfarin from albumin by acidic drugs. *Ann. N. Y. Acad. Sci., 179,* 213–225.

Shirley, H. F., and Kahn, J. P. A. 1958, Sleep disturbances in children. *Ped. Clin. N. Am., 5,* 629–643.

Teutsch, G., Mahler, D. L., Brown, C. R., Forrest, W. H., James, K. E., and Brown, B. W. 1975, Hypnotic efficacy of diphenhydramine, methapyrilene, and pentobarbital. *Clin. Pharm. Ther., 17,* 195–201.

Chapter Nine

USE OF DRUGS IN SPECIAL SYNDROMES: ENURESIS, TICS, SCHOOL REFUSAL, AND ANOREXIA NERVOSA

Lawrence M. Greenberg, M.D. & James H. Stephans, M.D.

INTRODUCTION

The special syndromes discussed in this chapter—enuresis, tics, school refusal, anorexia nervosa—have in common two characteristics: psychopharmacotherapy *may* play a role in their total psychiatric management; and the statements and recommendations for medications in this chapter are based on data obtained from *very few,* if any, adequately controlled and evaluated clinical studies.

In the psychopharmacological treatment, however, there are several general rules that warrant comment as an introduction:

1. Although the principal emphasis of this chapter is on psychopharmacological treatment, this by itself is not full or adequate treatment for these syndromes. As stressed by the authors of other chapters, (Campbell, ch. five; Cantwell, ch. six; Lucas, ch. seven), drug treatment must be preceded by a careful history, physical examination, and diagnostic formulation of the child, and then almost always accompanied by treatment approaches which deal with the child, family, and environment.

2. In addition to a thorough initial evaluation, there must be careful follow-up examinations. Certainly very careful and regular examinations are necessary not only to determine the efficacy of treatment but also to reduce the incidence and severity of side effects.

3. It is advisable to stop medication as soon as possible. Except for the Gilles

de la Tourette syndrome, the syndromes described here require relatively brief periods of treatment with medication.

These symptoms rarely present as emergencies, and initially high doses of medication are not necessary, the exception being when anorexia nervosa presents with life-threatening cachexia. Then medical treatment is indicated as a priority to the psychopharmacological treatment.

The special syndromes are presented in a similar format. A definition of the symptom or syndrome and clarification of the various terminologies in common usage are provided. Definition of pathology from normality is often a very difficult task, particularly in children who are undergoing rapid developmental and growth changes. It is equally difficult to distinguish among the parent's and child's chief complaints, the child's deviant behavior, and the actual target symptoms to be treated with medication. In addition to the primary emphasis on the psychopharmacological treatment of these symptoms, other aspects (incidence, natural history, and postulated etiologies) are considered briefly and references provided for readers seeking further details.

We emphasize the selection of the target symptom in order to initiate correct psychopharmacological treatment and assess the response to this treatment. For each symptom or syndrome the array of therapeutic compounds currently recommended is listed, and the relative merits, dosage ranges, side effects, treatment duration, follow-up frequency, and laboratory monitoring are reviewed. We recognize the generally unspoken controversy between two different methods of calculating the doses in children: milligram per kilogram and age-dependent doses. We use the milligram per kilogram approach for infants and young children in whom highly toxic levels may be readily encountered. However, consistent with the accepted procedures for the use of antiepileptic medications, we favor the age-dependent approach for medication treatment in school-aged and adolescent patients.

ENURESIS

Enuresis is the most common of the symptoms reviewed in this chapter, and is presented as the reference symptom to illustrate the general problems that are encountered to some degree in all the others. These problems include imprecise diagnostic definitions; difficulty distinguishing among pathological symptoms, presenting complaints, and age-appropriate behaviors; selection of particular target symptoms to be treated; and appropriate monitoring of the psychopharmacological treatment. We are limiting this discussion to involuntary wetting since voluntary wetting is rarely, if ever, treated with medications.

A vast yet contradictory medical literature pertaining to enuresis presents clearly divergent opinions and recommendations. The primary-care physician receives very different advice from the three medical specialties usually involved in the investigation and treatment of enuresis: urology, pediatrics, and child psychiatry. The urological literature emphasizes the presence and surgical correction of structural entities, the pediatric literature emphasizes relevant child-rearing techniques with use of a wetness detector alarm or psychoactive medication, and the psychiatric literature emphasizes the psychological abnormalities in the child and parents and recommends psychotherapy.

There are serious difficulties in defining the term *enuresis*. The Greek derivation of the word translates best perhaps as "surrounding oneself in one's own urine." The term has been used to indicate the wetting of bedclothes, and elaborated to include nocturnal enuresis or night wetting and diurnal enuresis or day wetting. Since nocturnal enuresis or night wetting may involve different levels of sleep as well as the waking state (Ritvo, Ornitz, Gottlieb, Poussaint, Maron, Ditman, and Blinn, 1969), arousal, nonarousal, and waking enuresis are also differentiated from each other. In the interests of clarity and parsimony, the simple descriptive terms, day wetting and night wetting, are used in this chapter, although we recognize the advantages of having more finely graduated and etiologically differentiated categories of enuresis.

Among the variables to be considered in establishing the diagnosis of enuresis, the age of the child is extremely important. In infancy, day and night wetting are normal behaviors; by adult age they are clearly pathological. Some authors rather arbitrarily use the occurrence of wetting after three years of age as indicative of pathology, while others suggest that wetting at seven years or even at twelve years of age may be a variation of normal (Forsythe and Redmond, 1974; Oppel, Harper, and Rider, 1968).

There is general agreement about the natural history of night and day wetting. McKendry and Stewart (1974), and Forsythe and Redmond (1974) report that 10–15 percent of children (especially males) past the age of five years continue to wet, and Oppel et al. (1968) find that 10 percent of seven-year-olds and 3 percent of twelve-year-olds continue to wet. Forsythe and Redmond additionally state that from five to sixteen years of age there is an annual spontaneous cure rate of 14–16 percent, and that 3 percent of the wetting children continue to wet past the age of twenty years. To establish meaningful age guidelines, we assume that most children in average expectable environments do cease involuntary day wetting by age five and involuntary night wetting by age six. We also assume that, in general, boys persist in wetting longer than do girls.

An important distinction is made between primary and secondary wetting (Forsythe and Redmond, 1974). Primary wetting refers to continual wetting since birth without a dry period in which bladder control was achieved. Secondary wetting refers to a relapse or recurrence of wetting after a period of dryness or bladder control. However, there is difficulty even with these apparently simple categories. Various definitions of the "dry period" are used, and parents often optimistically consider even a period as short as one week as the equivalent of having achieved bladder control. We require a minimum period of one month to assume true bladder control. One group of investigators (Oppel et al., 1968) report that over 90 percent of the relapsers or secondary wetters had dry periods which lasted six months or more. They cite this as evidence to support the popular and rather common-sense belief that secondary enuresis is not the result of congenital urinary abnormality. Therefore, if secondary wetting can be established by history, there is little reason to suspect any congenital pathology of the urinary system. There seems to be general agreement (Forsythe and Redmond, 1974; Oppel et al., 1968) that approximately one-quarter of all wetters are of the secondary or relapsed type. In addition, one group of authors (Oppel et al., 1968) suggests that parents of older children are apt to forget or at least fail to mention the occurrence of a significantly long dry interval in the past.

In most cases of primary wetting there does appear to be a physiological abnormality consisting of premature, involuntary, and uncontrollable bladder contractions with even small amounts of bladder fluid (McLellan, 1939). In these cases, urgency to urinate is a prominent symptom and wetting results. We view wetting beyond the age of six as a developmental delay and wetting after age twelve to be a developmental deviation.

The frequency of wetting is an important factor since the results of treatment often are reflected in a decrease rather than a cessation of wetting. Various authors have used frequencies of occurrence ranging from at least twice a week, once a month, or even so vague as all children mentioned by their mothers as bed wetting. In our experience the majority of children referred for evaluation because of enuresis wet frequently if not almost daily. The children who wet infrequently usually have significant environmental or situational problems contributing to if not causing the enuresis.

Day wetting is seriously neglected in the literature. The few articles that do consider day wetting either treat it as a variation of night wetting, or combine day and night wetting under the misnomer of diurnal wetting without attaching any etiological or prognostic significance to it. However, Forsythe and Redmond (1974) report that 13 percent of their series of combined day- and night-wetting cases continue to have day wetting after the night wetting ceases. This observation, along with the report of Ritvo et al. (1969) that 10 percent of their small series of night wetters actually are awake at the time of wetting, raises a question whether this type of wetting might sometimes be voluntary in origin. This runs contrary to the usual description of enuresis as "involuntary" (McKendry and Stewart, 1974).

A complete history and physical examination, including observation of the micturition process, are basic elements in the evaluation process. In addition to obtaining the details of the presenting complaint and clarifying the issues above, precipitating stresses as well as concurrent psychiatric disorders can be detected by history. (Parenthetically, the authors have had previously undiagnosed psychotic children referred because of enuresis.) We use a standardized history form to obtain basic factual information so as to allow sufficient time to explore such issues as the parents' attitudes toward toilet training, the child's attitudes toward his wetting, and the types of treatment that have been attempted. As discussed later in this chapter, a successful intervention often can be achieved simply by proper education.

Although the incidence of urinary tract problems is low even in cases of primary wetting, the majority must be approached with the recognition that wetting can be due to strictly organic causes. Urinary tract infections are an occasional cause of wetting, particularly in female children. Urinalysis and, if indicated, a urine culture can quickly resolve any question of infection. In adolescents, gonococcal urethritis can cause urinary strictures resulting in hesitancy, overflow incontinence, and dribbling. The history is of primary importance here, and if there is a possibility of exposure, appropriate diagnostic tests and urological evaluation are indicated.

Congenital abnormalities of the urinary tract are very uncommon. Forsythe and Redmond (1974) state that in 530 children examined with IVP and an additional 830 patients evaluated with very selective use of IVP, the incidence of an organic cause for wetting was less than one percent. A functionally decreased bladder size has been reported by many investigators (Troup and Hodgson, 1971), and it is widely reported that the functional size of the bladder increases with adequate treatment of the wetting. Neurological abnormalities should be ruled out by careful history of the developmental milestones as well as the screening neurological examination including sensory examination of the perineum. Congenital abnormalities of the spine rarely present with wetting as the initial difficulty, and would be ruled out by careful inspection of the skin over the spinal areas and the neurological examination. We recommend that radiological investigations be limited to those patients for whom there is a strong suspicion of organic pathology, or who fail to respond to adequate treatment.

If these diagnostic procedures are followed, and no medical illness is found, we assume that the wetting is due to inadequate or improper toilet-training techniques or psychogenic problems and do not pursue further diagnostic studies. The recommendation of some urologists (Arnold and Ginsburg, 1973) that there are "established or potentially obstructive genital urinary lesions in all children with persistent diurnal wetting systems" is contradictory to the facts and untenable.

The most common group of wetters is the primary type. Typically, the child is a member of a nondisrupted family, with or without a family history of wetting, with entirely normal developmental milestones, good general health, and without sleep or behavior disorders. A wide range of parental attitudinal problems can be described. At one extreme, the parents may be overly concerned, particularly with young children, and may have prematurely instituted a variety of popular procedures such as restricting evening fluid intake, emphasizing complete voiding prior to bedtime, placing the child on the toilet while asleep or awakening the child during the night to urinate. These procedures generally are both harmless and ineffective, although placing the sleeping child on the toilet could conceivably reinforce night wetting by teaching the child to urinate while asleep. Often the parents progress along a sequence of ineffective and inconsistent home remedies to the point where their own frustration leads them to react in anger, with loss of privileges, spankings, and verbal threats or humiliations. The child soon may develop a high level of anxiety with feelings of guilt and anger. At the other extreme of attitudes, the parents seem completely unconcerned about the wetting, and school officials, other parents, or even the child insist that the matter be brought to medical attention. This child usually is older and has little anxiety or guilt about the wetting except that related to teasing and taunting by peers. Interestingly, with both extremes of parental attitudes, it is common for the child to awaken upon wetting, then awaken the parents who change the bed clothes and the child's clothes. In one case an eight-year-old girl would awaken the family with yells for help and then get into the bed with her father while the mother changed the wet bed clothes. After awakening not only her own family, but also the author's family the first night of a camping trip, the problem dramatically ceased when told very clearly that she was no longer allowed to wake anyone up.

The appropriate treatment in these types of cases is, of course, reeducation of parents and child regarding bladder training. Three particularly important points need to be emphasized. First, the wetting is not an illness nor a willful act of defiance and, whatever the child's age, it is a relatively common occurrence. Second, it does not hurt the child physically or psychologically to lie in bed clothes that are wet with urine. (Mattresses are easily protected with a variety of waterproof covers.) Third, parental attention (either positive or negative) to wetness and dryness should be minimized, and the child should take complete charge of any necessary changing of wet clothes.

The second group of wetters has a secondary type of wetting, but otherwise a similar constellation of characteristics as the first group. The same investigation and intervention to modify the attitudes of the parents and children are necessary.

However, in these cases a thorough attempt must be made to identify the precipitating factor(s). The most common psychological stress related to the recurrence of wetting is the birth of a sibling; other precipitating situations include marital problems, starting school, death of a pet, and moving. Occasionally, secondary enuresis is the only symptom of a reactive depression. It is important that these precipitating events be identified both to parents and children, and that parents and physicians be instructed in supportive ways of helping the child deal with the loss or problem. Psychotherapy, individual or family, is indicated if reassurance and support does not help. Incidentally, it seems quite significant that when the reeducation and the psychotherapy techniques fail with this group of wetters, they show by far the best response to antidepressant medication treatment of any group. They seem to respond better to medication than to the alarm technique, discussed below.

In the third, and smallest, group of wetters a behavior disorder is present in addition to the wetting which can be of either the primary or secondary type. Often, this group of wetters has physically abusive parents who have angrily overreacted to the child's wetting. The children may become very angry and impulsive, with poor peer socialization, poor school performance, and occasionally destructiveness, cruelty to animals, and firesetting. This group of wetters requires a more intensive type of psychotherapeutic intervention.

It is difficult to evaluate the many variables that influence the success or failure of a therapeutic intervention. Certainly, motivation and consistency are critical factors. As an illustration of the incredible array of obstacles that can be encountered, a reeducation process almost failed because the parents of a seven-year-old girl had just purchased a large expensive bed which the child could not move away from the wall in order to change the sheets. Somehow the parents were unable to devise a temporary solution for the problem. If the family's performance is less than satisfactory, or if there are serious psychological problems which must be dealt with, it may be best to persevere with the reeducative techniques for several months. If the parents and the child appear to be using the counseling well, but the wetting continues after one month, we advise adding medication to the treatment. An important factor in the decision to move on to additional treatment modalities is the loss of hope.

After an unsuccessful reeducative attempt, the next intervention is medication. Modern psychopharmacological treatment of wetting involves the use of the tricyclic antidepressant medications. A host of medicants and medications have been prescribed for wetting, dating back at least to 1500 B.C. (Glicklich, 1951) and proceeding on into relatively modern times. Anticholinergics, amphetamine-like medications, and minor and major tranquilizers all have been recommended on the basis of studies of varying quality and reliability. It is safe to say that these medications are all useless in the treatment of wetting (Blackwell and Currah,

1973; Forsythe and Redmond, 1974). There is some valid evidence that the monoamine oxidase inhibitor type of antidepressant medication may be effective (Frommer, 1967, 1968), but in comparison with the tricyclic antidepressants, they are associated with a much higher risk of serious side effects and are not indicated or discussed further in this chapter.

The target symptom to be treated with medication is the wetting, and two treatment limitations are recognized. First, the tricyclics commonly produce a dramatic decrease in the frequency of wetting, but much less often a total cessation. This can be a source of disappointment to the parents, but with careful explanations and preparation before starting treatment, parents can be quite satisfied with a reduction in the frequency of wetting when complete cure does not result from treatment. Second, temporary use of the tricyclics often does not result in a permanent improvement. Ever since MacLean (1960) published the first article on the use of tricyclics in the treatment of wetting, and commented that the wetting often relapses as soon as the medication is stopped, this has been a consistent finding in the large majority of treated patients in all studies. As a result of these two limitations on the effectiveness of tricyclic treatment, there are ongoing debates and contradictory studies regarding the relative efficacy of the various tricyclic antidepressants, the dosages to be used, the time and frequency of administration, the duration of the treatment, the related question of repeated courses of treatment, and, finally, the question of turning to alternate forms of treatment, such as the wetness-detector alarm system and hypnotherapy. These questions are dealt with in turn.

Parenthetically, we hope that the prognostic significance of the emotional status of the child and the parents has been adequately stressed. If the poor self-esteem, depression, and acting out have persisted sufficiently long to become characterologically fixed, the treatment of the wetting is a relatively minor consideration. Since the antidepressants are not very effective in the treatment of childhood depression, psychotherapeutic treatment is necessary in these cases.

Of the various tricyclic antidepressant medications, imipramine was the first available and was the tricyclic used by MacLean (1960) in his pioneering study. Although it has become the prototype medication in the treatment of wetting, all of the tricyclic antidepressants appear to have a comparable beneficial effect in the treatment of wetting. Claims of superiority for one compound or another in the treatment of wetting have not been substantiated. As a general rule, imipramine has been the drug of choice, since clinicians are more familiar with its toxicity and dosages. However, if a sleep disturbance is encountered as a side effect, amitriptyline could be prescribed since it has a mild sedative effect. In the event of a therapeutic failure with imipramine, it is rather unlikely that any of the other tricyclics would be successful, but a trial with one of the other tricyclics might be advisable.

The mechanism of action of tricyclic antidepressants in the treatment of wetting is not understood. Several theories have been proposed and each has supporting but inconclusive data. The tricyclics do have anticholinergic side effects, including urinary retention. However, atropine-like or anticholinergic medications that are considerably more potent than the tricyclics have no significant effect on wetting (Blackwell and Currah, 1973; Forsythe and Redmond, 1974; Petersen, Anderson, and Hansen, 1974).

A second postulated mechanism of action for the tricyclics is via a change in the level of sleep. Although recent studies nearly conclusively demonstrate that night wetting can occur at any level of sleep and even while the patient is lying awake in bed (Ritvo et al., 1969), it is postulated that the tricyclics decrease the depth of sleep in certain subjects (Ritvo, Ornitz, LaFranchi, and Walter, 1967). There appeared to be two different patterns in this group of seven boys with primary enuresis. The first group involved subjects who had wetting associated with the awake state or with evidence of arousal on the all-night EEG tracings. This group also was characterized by the presence of other neurotic symptoms or behavior disorders, considerable family distress, and the occurrence of wetting late at night, often just prior to arising, and responded rather poorly to tricyclic treatment. The second group consisted of patients with predominantly nonarousal enuresis. Wetting occurred during the deeper stages of sleep with no evidence of arousal on the all-night EEG. These patients were characterized by minimal evidence of maladjustment and family concern about wetting, a history of frequent and heavy wetting relatively early in the evening, a frequently positive family history of wetting, and a much better response to imipramine treatment. Their parents also described them as being extremely deep sleepers. Although one might postulate that imipramine acts either by decreasing the depth of sleep or increasing the frequency of arousal phenomena prior to wetting, EEG studies fail to corroborate these predictions. The observed EEG changes with imipramine are an increased latency from sleep onset until the occurrence of the first REM phase, increased amount of stage two sleep, a decreased amount of stage one REM sleep and no alteration in the combined stage three-four sleep time. The authors (Ritvo et al., 1967) emphasize that their conclusions are based on a small sample and are hypothetical.

A third postulated mechanism of action for imipramine is the placebo effect, since some of the early double-blind studies following MacLean's report did not demonstrate significant effects. Some discussion of this hypothesis is warranted since it illustrates the difficulty in interpreting drug research. Blackwell and Currah (1973) suggested that a placebo response was either absent or negligible in all studies with an adequate baseline obtained prior to initiation of treatment. They concluded that the baseline obtained from the parents' history very commonly exaggerated the frequency of wetting, and that this accounted for the frequently reported placebo effects. However, of the studies they cited, all but one involved institutionalized patients (probably with other significant pathology), and the exception included an unusual double crossover design which could have minimized the placebo effect. Three of the seven studies they cited in institutionalized patients actually did have a relatively small but still statistically significant placebo response. We would agree that there is a definite placebo response, probably in the range reported by Petersen et al. (1974) of 31 percent, but we doubt that the placebo effect is the sole mechanism of action for imipramine.

The fourth mechanism of action proposed for imipramine is its antidepressant effect. Blackwell and Currah (1973) discount this possibility on the basis that the time course of action is much too rapid to be an antidepressant effect. Whereas in adults it takes at least ten days before an antidepressant effect appears, in children the response of wetting to the tricyclics occurs as soon as three to four days and usually within seven days. However, this argument is negated by the more recent findings of Perel (1975) that children reach a steady-state level of tricyclics in the blood much more rapidly than do adults. Perhaps the most enlightening study regarding mode of action is that of Petersen et al. (1974), comparing the effects of placebo, a pure anticholinergic medication, imipramine and imipramine-N-oxide (a new imipramine derivative presumably free of any anticholinergic effect). The results of the anticholinergic medication were equal to that of the placebo. Imipramine-N-oxide reduced the frequency of night wetting to 78 percent, and imipramine to 58 percent, of the placebo level. They concluded that the antidepressant effect did play a major role in the treatment of wetting, and that the anticholinergic effect contributed additionally, but only when added to the antidepressant effect.

It is very difficult to compare studies of tricyclic treatment in wetting because of the widely different evaluation procedures used by different authors (Blackwell and Currah, 1973). Certainly clinical judgment of efficacy is influenced by parental expectations for a total cessation of wetting and their disappointment with only a decrease in the frequency (Forsythe and Merit, 1969). Even excluding the overly optimistic and pessimistic reports, results vary from a high of 40 percent (Meadow, 1974) and 60 percent (Poussaint and Ditman, 1965) to a low of 10–20 percent (Blackwell and Currah, 1973) of patients becoming totally dry within one month of treatment. If only the secondary enuretics are considered, the response is considerably better (Shaffer, 1973; Shaffer, Costello, and Hill, 1968). However, estimates of the number of these patients who remain dry even shortly after cessation of the medication range from only 10 percent (Milner and Hills, 1968) to 30 percent (Yodfat, 1966).

If decrease in the frequency of wetting is considered a successful response, the results of imipramine treatment are considerably better. Many reports over the past decade suggest that the frequency of enuresis is reduced to between 56 and

79 percent of the frequency while on placebo (Petersen et al., 1974). Again, if only secondary wetters are considered, there is evidence that total improvement could be obtained and be superior to the wetness alarm system (Kolvin, Garside, Taunch, Currah, and McNay, 1973).

The methods of prescribing tricyclic antidepressants in wetters vary widely, with contradictory recommendations in the literature for dosages, the time of administration, and the duration of treatment, and divergent opinions about the onset of action, the side effects, and their severity (Blackwell and Currah, 1973).

MacLean (1960) arbitrarily chose and prescribed 25 mg. for children under twelve years of age and 50. mg for older children at bedtime. Subsequently, and unfortunately too frequently in drug studies, most of the researchers have continued to use the same doses. Further complicating dosage recommendations is the ongoing controversy among advocates for the different methods of administration (mg./kmg., mg./surface area, and gradual increments). Few significant differences in responses to dosage levels have been reported; however, dosage ranges have generally been limited to 25 to 75 mg./day. Some clinicians have recommended adult-level dosages for children as young as six to eight years of age, since the central nervous system grows and matures at a much faster rate than any other system of the body. Many clinicians have been hesitant to use "high" levels of medication and prescribe on the basis of weight, size, or age. The report (Saraf, Klein, Gittelman-Klein, and Groff, 1974) of a fatality perhaps secondary to a high level of imipramine lends support to a more conservative approach. Further, Perel (1975) has recently reported that the metabolism of tricyclics in the liver (a relatively large organ for body size in children) appears to be faster in children than in adults. Thus, not only do blood levels of tricyclics rise more rapidly than in adults, there is also a higher level of toxic metabolites than in adults. Perel recommends that these medications be started in small doses, be given frequently, and kept at lower levels than ordinarily used with adults. We recommend starting dosages of 25 mg. for children under twelve and 50 mg. for older children, but with considerable flexibility in adjusting the dose if an adequate response is not obtained. We recommend gradually increasing the dose from the initial level if no response is reached in the first week until levels of between 50–75 mg. are reached in children under twelve and levels of 100 mg. of imipramine are reached in older children.

Although traditionally administered at bedtime, later studies have suggested (but not clearly established) that for wetting occurring primarily before midnight an early evening administration is more effective than a bedtime dosage. It may be valuable to consider the two most probable mechanisms of action of the tricyclic medications, the anticholinergic and the antidepressant effects as described above. The antidepressant effect requires a minimum of three to four days to become apparent. Therefore, this aspect of the therapeutic effect of the tricyclics would not be dependent upon the time of administration. However, the anticholinergic effect of imipramine has been shown to peak three hours after administration, but to persist for 72 hours (Blackwell and Currah, 1973). Since this action of the tricyclics would be very dependent upon the time of administration, a flexible approach should be used. If there is day wetting as well as night wetting, three-times-a-day doses should be used. If the wetting occurs prior to midnight, a late afternoon dose should be used; if the wetting is after midnight, a bedtime dose should be used.

Recommendations for duration of treatment with tricyclics vary from the usual of a minimum of one month to "prolonged and continuous treatment" (Lake, 1968). We recommend that if a satisfactory response is reached within the first month of treatment, the medication should be discontinued after one month, and restarted for a second month if the child relapses. The decision to treat for a third month or a more protracted course must be made on an individual basis. On the other hand, if during the initial month of treatment no satisfactory response is attained, it would seem reasonable to continue the treatment for eight weeks with adjustments in time of administration and dosage level. After failure to achieve a satisfactory response with tricyclic medications, alternate methods of treatment, alarm systems, or rarely hypnotherapy should be considered. As a general rule, we recommend limiting tricyclic treatment to six months.

Few side effects are reported with these doses and durations of tricyclics. The most commonly reported side effects of imipramine are difficulty getting to sleep and occasional nightmares. Also reported are change in daytime mood with increased irritability and restlessness. Although dizziness is described, it appears to occur as frequently with placebo as with imipramine. Mild anorexia has been noted. Paralytic ileus has been reported in one case (Milner and Hills, 1968) and an epileptic seizure in one case (Fisher, Murray, Walley, and Kiloh, 1963). Shaffer et al. (1968) reported the development of an acute peptic ulcer in one case, but it was considered coincidental (Blackwell and Currah, 1973). Reports of side effects with amitriptyline have been extremely rare and have generally been similar to the side effects from imipramine. As with all medications, idiosyncratic reactions can be encountered even with low doses, and the physician must continue to observe the patient closely. The most serious side effect reported has been changes in cardiac conduction with arrhythmia. Saraf et al. (1974) reported the first sudden death (in a child) with high dosages of imipramine possibly due to an arrhythmia. Fortunately, the study by Martin and Zaug (1975) failed to demonstrate EKG changes in children receiving low dosages of imipramine. There are two recent reports, however, (Greenberg and Yellin, 1975; Saraf et al., 1974) that quite surprisingly note that hypertension occasionally may be induced by imipramine (in the treatment of hyperactivity).

The following procedure is suggested in initiating and following up tricyclic treatment for wetting. At the initial evaluation, the family and patient should be seen. A thorough history and physical examination should be carried out as described earlier. The actual micturition should be observed either by the physician or by a trained nurse, and a urinalysis obtained. If the urinalysis reveals excessive white cells, a urine culture is in order. If either the urine culture or stream are abnormal, appropriate workup for organic lesions is indicated. If evidence of neurological, spinal, or psychiatric illness is present, further evaluation is indicated. Treatment should be initiated as described in the above paragraphs, starting with toilet-training reeducation and, when indicated, psychotherapy. If there is an inadequate response to these efforts, and the decision to undertake treatment with medication is made following the guidelines in the preceding paragraphs, treatment with imipramine should be started. The initial dose is 25 mg. for children under twelve and 50 mg. for children over twelve years. If the wetting is before midnight, the dosage can be given in the later afternoon, and if wetting is after midnight, medication can be given prior to bedtime. The family and the patient should be given a list of possible side effects with instructions to call immediately should any of them occur. If there are no complications, the family and the patient are seen one week later when the blood pressure is checked, and response as well as side effects are determined. If there is not a satisfactory response within two weeks, the medication gradually should be increased to 50 mg. in children under twelve and 75 mg. in children over twelve. The patient should be seen again one month after initiating tricyclic medication. At that point, if the result is satisfactory, the medication should be tapered and stopped over a two-week period. The patient and family may be discharged at that point with instructions to return for another trial of medication should the wetting recur. Routine follow-up with blood counts and liver tests seem of little value since treatment with medication is relatively short term, and these tests are not sufficiently sensitive to predict the idiosyncratic reactions.

If there is a complete failure to respond to medication, a wetness detector and hypnosis may be considered. Although these treatments are beyond the scope of this book, brief comments are indicated. The conditioning with a buzzer system is widely used in Great Britain, with up to an 80-percent success rate for complete dryness reported (Turner, 1973). However, the author warns that there may be a relapse rate of one-third. Techniques of treatment with this apparatus are not so simple as one might imagine (Dische, 1973). The child must have matured to an age of responsibility adequate to handle the apparatus (Meadow, 1974). The treatment is not entirely benign. During its early use in Britain in the late 1950s, an incidence of skin rash of 20 percent was reported. Subsequently it has been realized that seriously infected ulcerations can occur (Meadow, 1973) when the buzzer alarm fails to awaken the child who continues to lie in the wet bedclothes with the current flowing between the electrodes. As a result, the British National

Health Service of 1968 issued a set of basic safety requirements, operating requirements, and recommendations for including a light along with the alarm.

TICS

In this category the primary focus is on one particular group, Gilles de la Tourette's syndrome. We do not use nor recommend pharmacotherapy as routine treatment of common tics. Certainly, when tics are so severe as to be incapacitating, medications can be used to decrease the level of anxiety. We do, however, discuss common tics in this section to differentiate them from the Tourette's syndrome.

For the past hundred years, this rare syndrome, known as Gilles de la Tourette's syndrome or Maladie des tics (Mahler, 1943), has attracted a great deal of interest. In spite of its rarity (prevalence estimates vary from 0.25 to 4 cases/100,000 population, Woodrow, 1974). there are many reasons why it deserves emphasis in a book on psychopharmacology in childhood and adolescence: First, onset occurs usually during childhood with a mean age of seven years and a range of two to eighteen years with 85 percent of the cases beginning before age ten (Woodrow, 1974). Second, it commonly is undiagnosed or misdiagnosed for unreasonably long periods of time. In one study of thirty-four patients, the interval between onset of symptoms and diagnosis of Tourette's syndrome was 9.0 years with a range of 0.2 years to 54 years (Shapiro, Shapiro, and Wayne, 1972a). Third, it has been demonstrated nearly conclusively that the treatment of choice is psychopharmacological. Fourth, there is increasing evidence (Shapiro, Shapiro, Wayne, Clarkin, and Brunn, 1973c; Lucas, 1970) that prompt and proper use of psychopharmacological treatment can enable the child psychiatrist to utilize other modalities of treatment, such as individual, family, and group psychotherapy and special education techniques to prevent the emergence of secondarily derived maladaptive personality characteristics or traits.

For several reasons this unusual illness has attracted a great deal of medical attention, including the bizarre qualities of the symptoms, the problems of differential diagnosis, the concern about biological versus psychogenic origins, and, after decades of unsuccessful treatment attempts and continued uncertainty about the natural course of the illness itself, a strikingly efficacious treatment now available. Now that apparently effective and relatively safe techniques of psychopharmacological treatment for this disorder are well defined, it becomes increasingly important to diagnose the syndrome earlier, employ more sophisticated methods for sorting out the primary and secondary symptoms, and utilize a full array of therapeutic techniques to prevent emergence of the secondary symptoms.

Correct diagnosis of a fully developed case of Tourette's syndrome is not difficult. The irregularly repeated, sudden, almost violent, involuntary muscle movements (very rarely organized into an obscene appearing gesture) combined with the equally explosive and usually simultaneous vocalizations (frequently organized into a recognizable word) can be diagnosed at a distance. In approximately half of the patients, the vocalizations are obscene, giving rise to the pathognomonic coprolalia. The imitative motor and verbal features (echopraxia and echolalia), which are probably overemphasized, occur infrequently and are not necessary for the diagnosis.

In its earlier stages, however, this illness can be extremely difficult to recognize. Statistics on misdiagnosis of the syndrome attest to this difficulty (Shapiro, Shapiro, Wayne, and Clarkin, 1972b). The importance of a precise diagnosis is increased by the serious hazards of an error in either direction: If the diagnosis is not made and appropriate psychopharmacological treatments not started, the patient (almost always a child) can be subject to irreversible personality changes relating to his own and his peers' reactions to his involuntary movements and vocalizations. If the diagnosis is incorrect, the patient will be subjected to longterm treatment with potent, potentially harmful medication. For these reasons, we recommend that whenever the question of this illness arises, the diagnosis and institution of treatment be carried out only with appropriate consultation, preferably at a tertiary treatment center.

Two characteristics of the illness contribute to early diagnostic difficulties. The first is the usually slow, insidious onset in childhood, as first noted by Gilles de la Tourette. The second feature, the waxing and waning course of the illness with remissions and relapses, was not recognized by Gilles de la Tourette. He considered the symptoms to be progressive and permanent.

The diagnostic problem that is probably the most common and difficult to avoid is differentiating the earliest symptoms of this syndrome from the common, usually transient, and benign tics of childhood. The age of onset (the early school-age years) and the most common initial sign (motor tic involving the eye lids or other facial musculature) are the same. Both types of tics are frequently accompanied by some emotional disturbance, often of an affective nature with anxiety, depression, or aggressive acting out (Corbett, Mathews, Connell, and Shapiro, 1969). Tics in childhood are quite common, occurring in 5 percent of seven-year-old children (Kellmer Pringle, Butler, and Davie, 1967) with a high rate of spontaneous recovery, ranging from 50 percent (Torup, 1962) to 80 percent (Corbett et al., 1969). To complicate matters, the latter authors suggest that the Tourette's syndrome is "simply the more severe presentation of the tic syndrome.'' In contrast, Brunn and Shapiro (1972) emphasize the diagnostic differences between common tics and Tourette's syndrome. We suggest the following guidelines: 1. The ordinary tic syndrome usually reaches a peak between five to ten years of age and begins to resolve at puberty. Tourette's syndrome has a more waxing and waning course but usually becomes more severe at puberty. 2. The common tic syndrome usually is limited to the muscles of the face and sometimes the neck and shoulders. Progressive involvement of the arm, hand, and particularly the lower extremities would be considered a strong indication of an evolving Tourette's syndrome. 3. Common tic syndrome movements are usually rather simple in nature, closely fitting Kanner's (1957) definition as "quick, sudden, and frequently repeated movement of circumscribed movements of muscles, having no apparent purpose.'' On the other hand, the movements in the Tourette's syndrome frequently become more complex and organized with a bizarre or violent quality. 4. Later development of involuntary vocalizations, intelligible or not, should be considered strongly indicative of Tourette's syndrome. 5. Involuntary utterances of obscene words (in the patient's native language) are considered pathognomonic for Tourette's syndrome. 6. If the vocalizations or lower extremity involuntary movements are the initial presenting signs, Tourette's syndrome should be considered the most likely diagnosis. 7. Imitative behaviors, echolalia or echopraxia, although extremely rare in the early phases of the illness, again make the diagnosis of Tourette's syndrome more likely.

Differentiating between the common tic syndrome and Tourette's syndrome is a clinical process with little help from laboratory and psychological testing. However, evidence of organicity on psychological testing is found in approximately half of the Tourette's syndrome cases (Shapiro, Shapiro, Wayne, and Clarkin, 1973b). EEG's frequently have mild abnormalities but are not in any way diagnostic for Tourette's syndrome. Both groups of patients have a normal distribution in I.Q. tests and commonly experience emotional disturbances. Both groups are aggravated by anxiety, stress, tension, and fatigue and improve with relaxation. Tics do not occur during sleep although there is disagreement about the occurrence of Tourette tics during sleep (Chapel, 1970). Finally, both groups can have a positive family history.

Other illnesses also must be differentiated from this syndrome. Obsessive-compulsive neurosis can be confused with Tourette's syndrome. Although some of the more organized motor movements and intelligible verbalizations (in the syndrome) might appear to have a compulsive quality, they are quite clearly involuntary in nature, as opposed to the voluntary quality that is, by definition, necessary for a compulsion. Also, the Tourette patient's behavior lacks the truly organized quality of compulsive behavior. Occasionally the stereotype motor movements of a schizophrenic patient may superficially resemble the involuntary movements of Tourette's syndrome. However, careful assessment of the course and the clinical evaluation of the patient make this diagnosis apparent. There should be little difficulty in distinguishing the seemingly self-stimulatory movements of the autistic child and the impulsive, uncontrolled movements of the mentally retarded, brain-damaged child from the behavior of the Tourette's syndrome patient. Sydenham's Chorea occasionally presents a more difficult diagnostic problem. However, the prior history of rheumatic fever, positive in 75 percent of these patients, and the careful observation of the quality of the movements, should be helpful. A number of rare neurological illnesses, which frequently are progressive and fatal, might be confused with Tourette's syndrome during the earliest phases. However, neurological findings usually are prominent in these illnesses, but only "soft signs" of CNS malfunctioning are found in half of the patients (Brunn and Shapiro, 1972). Finally, the esoteric illnesses of Latah, Myriachit, and "the jumpers" could be confused with this syndrome. In fact, Gilles de la Tourette considered them to be the same illness except in different cultural settings. However, these other illnesses clearly do not involve purely spontaneous, involuntary reactions, but instead are "startle reactions" to some external precipitant (Chapel, 1970).

The etiology of the syndrome is unknown. Unlike many other illnesses with as yet undiscovered etiologies, however, there is an especially tantilizing quality to the mystery of its origins. Since the involuntary movements of this syndrome seem to have much in common with other involuntary movement disorders with well-demonstrated neuropathology involving the basal ganglia, many people assume that there is a lesion to be detected. Even psychodynamically oriented authors such as Mahler, Luke, and Daltroff (1945) assume that there is most likely "a substratum of organic disease." However, autopsy examinations have been inconclusive, and occasional reports of pathology have not been replicated. Various encephalitic illnesses have been implicated, but cases with documented encephalitis are not considered to be true Gilles de la Tourette cases. For a review of the many neurophysiological theories, the reader is referred to the article by Corbin (1970).

The marked preponderance of cases in males over females (between 2:1 and 4:1) and known familial occurrence (Friel, 1973; Sanders, 1973) provide no definite evidence for a genetic component.

There is general agreement that psychological factors are involved in this disease, at least secondarily. The anxiety, depression, and feelings of rejection often seen in these children appear to be reactions to the teasing and jeering by their peers, and later become part of personality structure. Occasionally, more aggressive and sometimes antisocial behaviors occur. The evolution of the unintelligible vocalizations into intelligible words, often of obscene quality, commonly is held to be due to psychological factors. The obscene words generally involve references to sexual, urinary, or fecal functioning, and do not involve religious or ideological profanities. The argument that the obscene utterances could be on an organic basis, much as the organic aphasic patients retain only or regain first the obscene swear words, does not seem applicable here since the aphasic patient's obscenities are much less selective and circumscribed.

A more recent, unsubstantiated but very attractive etiological hypothesis presumes a biochemical abnormality of the neurotransmitter substances (Woodrow, 1974). Although there is no good evidence that either dopamine or norepinephrine metabolism is disturbed in patients with Tourette's syndrome, the very impressive benefit of haloperidol may well be the result of its effect on these two neurotransmitters.

Although there is little agreement about the etiology of this syndrome, there is consensus about the treatment. The treatment of choice is haloperidol. Omitting the overly optimistic and pessimistic reports, definite improvement can be obtained in 90 percent of the patients (Gold, Kline, and Winick, 1969; Shapiro et al., 1973c). Most authors (Abuzzahab, 1976; Shapiro et al., 1973c) agree that haloperidol should be started with low doses, 2 to 6 mg./day depending upon age, but rather rapidly increased to high levels until either the desired clinical improvement is reached or side effects occur which cannot be controlled without reducing the dosage. With older adolescents and adults, Shapiro et al. (1973c) and Abuzzahab (1976) report using doses up to 100–200 mg./day of haloperidol. In contrast, Lucas (1967) states that most of his patients have been treated adequately with 4–6 mg./day of haloperidol. Again, it is essential to weigh carefully the balance between the dangers of the illness and of the medication. Generally, extrapyramidal symptoms are not a deterrent to maintaining or increasing the medication unless the symptoms cannot be controlled by either an antiparkinsonism medication, diphenhydramine (Benadryl) or a combination of the two. For children twelve years of age and older, we treat the extrapyramidal symptoms with either benztropine mesylate (Cogentin) or trihexyphenidyl (Artane), 2 mg. at bedtime, or diphenhydramine (Benadryl), 25–50 mg. four times a day. With children under the age of twelve, the doses are approximately halved, and greater caution is used, often reducing the dosage level of haloperidol instead of continuing with the extrapyramidal medication. The extrapyramidal medication can be discontinued after three months since these symptoms usually cease during that interval.

Urinary retention may present a problem. In children over twelve years of age, the dosage of haloperidol does not need to be decreased since this symptom usually is a very temporary anticholinergic side effect which generally responds promptly to urecholine (5–15 mg. three times a day). Urethral catheterization is usually unnecessary in younger patients, since the likelihood of an obstructive retention is almost nonexistent. Constipation is an occasional transient side effect and should be treated symptomatically. Dry mouth and blurred vision are almost universal and transient side effects. They are not indications for altering the treatment, and careful explanation to the child and parents is essential to minimize apprehension and discomfort. Light sensitivity is another rare, but occasionally serious side effect that can be easily avoided. Patients on haloperidol should be warned about sensitivity to sunlight and advised to wear dark glasses and a sun screen type of sunburn lotion before going out into sunlight.

Although haloperidol is more effective overall, it is worth noting that in a few treatment failures, patients have shown a striking response to the high potency, low dosage phenothiazines, particularly fluphenazine. A newer antipsychotic agent, pimozide, reportedly a more specific dopamine neurotransmitter blocking agent with less anticholinergic and little norepinephrine blocking effects, shows some promise, but there is need for further clinical studies to find an effective agent with the fewest side effects (Abuzzahab, 1976).

Duration of the treatment is indefinite. Because treatment may be necessary for many years, even decades, it should be emphasized again that this is not a treatment that should be undertaken without due consideration and consultation. Once the desired therapeutic response has been achieved, there should be repeated attempts to establish medication at the lowest effective level. Shapiro (1970) reports that an average maintenance dose of 9 mg./day of haloperidol in his series of patients. Since the natural course of the illness is one of waxing and waning with occasional spontaneous remissions, we recommend that an attempt be made every three to six months to decrease the dosage. It is strongly recommended that the so-called "drug holiday" method of prescribing be instituted within the first six months of treatment or as soon as the dosage level of the patient has stabilized with the desired clinical effects. A "drug holiday" involves withdrawal of medication first one day, usually Sunday, and later two days a week.

Drug interactions are always important considerations. It is well documented that the barbiturates, perhaps some of the new nonbarbiturate hypnotics, and many of the anticonvulsant medications that have a barbiturate form as a breakdown product all interfere with the action of phenothiazines and haloperidol. Although there are many reports that phenothiazines and haloperidol lower the seizure threshold, initiation of seizures in patients with Tourette's syndrome treated with haloperidol has not been reported. Also benztropine and presumably other antiparkinsonism medications have been reported to decrease the antipsychotic effect of phenothiazines and haloperidol. Although clinical improvement in Tourette's syndrome has not been reported to be diminished by these antiparkinsonism medications, they should be reduced and discontinued as soon as possible.

Laboratory tests, specifically white blood counts, differentials, and liver function tests, have not proved very beneficial in early detection and prevention of liver and blood toxicity. Although liver toxicity from phenothiazines and halo-peridol is almost always reversible once the medication is terminated after jaundice is noted, and since an aplastic anemia is almost always irreversible when an early neutrocytopenia is detected after clinical signs occur, the only justification for performing these tests routinely is on a medical-legal basis.

Because of the efficacy of haloperidol and related compounds in the treatment of this illness, there is a new potential for effective psychotherapy with these patients. With younger patients and limited progression of the illness, there is an opportunity for prevention of secondary personality defects. At a later age, the psychotherapy promotes rehabilitation.

With careful assessment, early detection, prompt and proper initiation of psychopharmacological treatment, and full use of psychotherapeutic techniques, the treatment of this illness can be very successful.

SCHOOL REFUSAL

There is substantial literature concerning school phobia or school refusal. Most of this literature involves etiological formulations and treatment approaches stressing psychodynamic and occasionally behaviorist theoretical frameworks. Only recently have articles begun to appear dealing with this subject in biological and psychopharmacological terms (Frommer, 1967, 1968; Gittelman-Klein, 1975; Gittelman-Klein and Klein, 1973). For a review of the psychodynamic etiological and treatment theories, the reader is referred to the chapter on neurosis in childhood by Kessler (1972). For more specific examples of treatment interventions of a psychotherapeutic or counseling nature, the reader is referred to Skynner's article (1974).

If absences caused by actual physical illnesses are subtracted from the total of school absences, the remaining absences are generally labelled school avoidance. Beginning with the work of Johnson, Falstein, Szurek, and Svendsen (1941), a distinction has developed between school phobia and school truancy. Clinically the distinction often is quite straightforward; the school-phobic child usually is a shy, dependent, and often clinging child with obvious anxiety of a separation type associated with the mother, and when he avoids school, he spends the time at or near home. The school-truant child is much more independent and self-confident, exhibits little anxiety, is not really uncomfortable while at school but rather bored or scornful. When absent from school he usually is in the company of other truanting children who spend the time playing away from home and without the parents' knowledge. Family constellations are also strikingly different. The phobic child's parents usually manifest considerable psychopathology often centered about dependency needs, whereas the school truant's parents more frequently have disrupted marriages or significantly less concern and anxiety about the child.

Very early, Johnson et al. (1941) identified the significance of separation anxiety in school phobia and described the fear of separation as shared by both the mother and the child, with the mother's problem the primary one and the child's the secondary or induced one. Eisenberg (1958) and Hersov (1960) reaffirmed this finding, and a technique of treatment evolved which emphasized insistence on return of the child to school with a focus on psychotherapy for the child to overcome the separation anxiety, and for the mother to allow the child to become more independent. Malmquist (1965) emphasized the father's role as a contributor to the child's psychopathology of school phobia with greater emphasis placed on family therapy. (For an example of specific family therapy techniques, the reader is referred to the article by Berger, 1974). Sperling (1967) made a valuable contribution when she distinguished between two different types of school phobia. She attributed the first type, "induced school phobia," to a pathological parent-child relationship. The second type, "traumatic or common type of acute school phobia," was caused by a precipitating event that represented a danger to the child's ability to control reality (essentially the mother).

There has been a recent addition to the etiological formulations for school refusal, initiated first by Gittelman-Klein and Klein (1973). They suggest, based on the results of their initially empirical use of imipramine in treating school refusal, that there may be a pathological process intrinsic to the child, and "challenge the model which posits an extrinsic source of anxiety." Although this very provocative hypothesis has not been clearly substantiated, there certainly is some early supporting evidence for this theory (Berg, Marks, McGuire, and Lipsedge, 1974; Tyrer and Tyrer, 1974).

Whatever the ultimate etiology or etiologies may be, there are particularly important clinical and diagnostic features in the psychopharmacological treatment of school refusal:

1. Even in the presence of documented physical disease, often of a chronic nature, a psychogenic school refusal can be present and be related to the child's embarrassment over defective appearance or performance, teasing from other children, or easy fatigability. As has been noted by others (Lansky, Lowman, Vats, and Gyulay, 1975), this school refusal can be extremely refractory because of the parents' insistence that "it's all physical" and can have a severe effect on the quality of the sick child's life. A high index of suspicion certainly seems indicated in chronically ill children, even to the point of checking with school officials if there is some indication that the parents may be hiding this problem.

Early and intensive psychotherapeutic intervention is indicated, and in the authors' opinion if there is no response within a few weeks, psychopharmacological treatment should be instituted.

2. Considerable progress has been made in the identification and differentiation of subtle specific learning defects which in the past so often were missed or confused with mental retardation. It is becoming increasingly apparent that these subtle learning defects, as well as subtle auditory and visual defects can be a primary cause of school refusal. These should be considered during the evaluation of a case of school refusal so that the primary disturbance can be treated as effectively as possible.

3. The reality of school situations should be considered. Unfortunately, peer interactions today sometimes involve more than just bullying or teasing; terrorism, extortion for lunch money, and physical brutality do occur in the early grades. Racial prejudice and scapegoating are not unknown. The child's fears about school, until known to be otherwise, should be considered realistic and not phobic.

4. An operational definition of school refusal is difficult because there appears to be an intermediate group of children who attend school sporadically, never missing more than a few days at a time, but performing poorly and reporting high degrees of anxiety and discomfort at school. The authors feel that this group should be included with school refusals along with those who fit a more traditional definition of "staying away from school for at least two weeks with a great reluctance or fear about going back." (Berg et al., 1974.)

5. It seems evident, as Sperling (1967) first indicated, that there is more than one type of school refusal or school phobia. Her distinction between those with and those without a precipitating traumatic event is very pertinent. The more common precipitating events appear to be entrance into first grade and junior high school, and the incidence of school refusals is heavily clustered at ages five to eight and eleven to fourteen (Tyrer and Tyrer, 1974). Also there is evidence that onset of severe marital discord in the parents, death of a sibling, and impending departure of an older sibling from the family may precipitate school refusals. It seems evident that the precipitating event should be a major focus of the psychotherapy. Generally the presence of a precipitating event indicates a better prognosis. Particularly in the adolescent, the absence of a precipitating event at the onset of school refusal can be indicative of a more serious illness such as an emerging schizophrenic process.

6. In addition to the two groups identified by Sperling (1967), there appear to be other subgroups. Gittelman-Klein and Klein (1973) identified three subgroups: (1) children who completely refused school for at least two weeks and displayed manifest anxiety; (2) children with intermittent school attendance but severe separation anxiety; and (3) children who refused absolutely to go to school

for at least two weeks but had no evidence of any separation anxiety. Also it has been observed that some of the school-refusal children display different patterns of separation anxiety. Some children have a decrease of their anxiety only when they are in the actual presence of the mother, some are comfortable if they are in the home with or without the mothers, and others are comfortable as long as they stay within a certain distance of the home. Some children are comfortable at school as long as the mother is in close attendance, while others are not comfortable even when the mother is there. The significance of these various subtypes is uncertain at this time, but hopefully they will prove to have some prognostic and therapeutic value.

7. Age of onset of school refusal is a valid criterion for prediction of outcome. The prognosis is better when the onset is before eleven years of age (Kennedy, 1965; Rodriguez, Rodriguez, and Eisenberg, 1959; Warren, 1965), and there is evidence (Tyrer and Tyrer, 1974) that onset of school refusal after eleven years of age is more closely associated with adult neurosis.

8. Since Eisenberg's report in 1958 that school phobia appeared to be increasing in prevalence, there have been repeated suggestions that this may be the case; however, no detailed demographic statistics are available. Miller, Hampe, Barrett, and Noble (1971) reported a prevalence of school refusal of 1 percent of the general population of school children while Mitchell and Shepherd (1967) suggested that 5 percent of the general schoolchild population disliked being at school and this aversion was associated with refusal. School phobia is estimated to comprise about 5 percent of child psychiatric referrals. However, the Tyrer and Tyrer (1974) retrospective study indicates that only 28.6 percent of psychiatric adult patients who had a history of school refusal were referred to a psychiatric clinic. This fact combined with several reports (Gittelman-Klein and Klein, 1973; Berg et al., 1974; Tyrer and Tyrer, 1974) that there is a clear association of childhood school refusal with adult neurotic illness make it imperative that greater efforts be made to educate parents and school officials to initiate consultations for school refusals.

9. Although there appears to be a definite association between childhood school refusal and adult neurosis as cited above, there is often a trouble-free interval between the school phobia and the later adult neurosis. Thus, there is concern that actual return to school is not the critical treatment issue in school refusal. Instead, adequate management of all of the psychiatric problems is necessary.

While psychopharmacological treatment may be an important modality, it is not the primary or initial treatment modality in school refusal. The following procedure is suggested as optimum treatment based on current knowledge:

The initial treatment involves an intensive effort utilizing environmental maneuvers to help the child reenter school, combined with individual psychotherapy, parental counseling, and family psychotherapy as appropriate. The majority of children respond to this approach and only a small minority require psychopharmacological treatment. If there is no progress after two weeks of intensive treatment, the prognosis appreciably worsens, and psychopharmacological treatment should be initiated. Since this is not a life-threatening or malignant disorder, we recommend a relatively benign first stage of psychopharmacological treatment and consider use of a placebo or small, infrequent doses of a minor tranquilizer. The placebo response has been demonstrated to result in a 50-percent success rate in returning very refractory school-refusal patients to school (Gittelman-Klein and Klein, 1973). Alternatively, or if the placebo does not result in quick improvement within one to two weeks, low doses of a benzodiazepine could be utilized (Skynner, 1974), although most clinicians would choose to prescribe a tricyclic at this stage of the illness. If a medication like chlordiazepoxide is chosen, 5–10 mg. are given, usually one hour before school. A second dose during the noon hour may occasionally be necessary. To reduce the potential addicting characteristics of these medicines, no medication is given on nonschool days. The medicine is discontinued within two weeks after successful return of the child to school. If the child reports a recurrence of anxiety, the minor tranquilizer can be reinstituted as necessary for a second or even third two-week trial. If the patient then cannot be withdrawn from the medication, the minor tranquilizer should be discontinued, and the tricyclic antidepressants used.

Early reports (Gittelman-Klein and Klein, 1973) indicate a strikingly successful rate of response in a double-blind, placebo controlled study of the effects of imipramine in thirty-five school-phobic children, aged six to fourteen, who had not responded to two weeks of intensive psychotherapy. They reported no differences between placebo and imipramine in three weeks of treatment. However, after six weeks of treatment, the imipramine group had an 81-percent successful return to school by contrast to a 47-percent success with placebo. The psychiatrists' and the mothers' ratings of global improvement after six weeks of treatment were even more striking. The psychiatrists rated 73 percent of the imipramine-treated patients, but only 32 percent of the placebo patients as much improved. The mothers reported 87 percent of the imipramine patients, but only 42 percent of the placebo patients much improved. One interesting feature of this excellent study, the children's self-ratings, revealed that 100 percent of the imipramine-treated patients, but only 21 percent of the placebo patients reported much improvement.

The technique of prescribing tricyclic antidepressants for school refusal still remains uncertain. In their initial reports, Gittelman-Klein and Klein (1973) reported minimal side effects, primarily dry mouth, although using very high doses of imipramine. They subsequently have reported the death of a child on high-dose imipramine (Saraf et al., 1974). In addition there are two reports of significant hypertension induced in children receiving imipramine (Greenberg and Yellin, 1975). These clinical reports plus evidence of faster metabolism of imipramine in children with the resultant rapid build-up of potentially toxic metabolic products (Perel, 1975) compel caution. The advantages of tricyclic antidepressant treatment must be weighed carefully against the severity of the illness. Gittelman-Klein (1975) reported, "Many children require imipramine doses in the adult range (100–200 mg./day). However, a 200-mg. daily dose should not be exceeded in view of the possibility of severe effects at the upper limit of the adult dose used in depression." She also stated, "No child between the ages of six and fourteen responded to less than 75 mg./day in the experimental school phobic group"; however, among other children that she had treated clinically for separation anxiety without school phobia, low loses (25–50 mg./day) were effective in some cases. The key point made by the author is that "the age and size of the child do not provide clear guidelines for appropriate dose levels." She also stated that once-a-day (at night) doses appeared to be as effective as twice-a-day dosage schedules, and that after a treatment course of at least six weeks, there should be a tapering over a one-week period before discontinuation.

Although it would seem logical that any of the tricyclic antidepressants could be as effective in the treatment of school refusal, imipramine is the only tricyclic studied to date. We recommend twice-a-day administration because of Perel's findings (1975), plus the fact that a large bedtime dose occasionally interferes with sleep. A cautious dosage schedule is used, particularly in the first two weeks of treatment. Gittelman-Klein and Klein's schedule (1973) can be used as a guide: For the first three days, dosage should be limited to 25 mg./day regardless of age; for the next four days dosage should be limited to 50 mg./day. In the second week dosage should be limited to 75 mg./day regardless of age. After the second week if there has not been a satisfactory response to the lower doses, we recommend that medication be gradually increased to a daily maximum of 50 mg. twice a day for children between six and eight years of age and 75 mg. twice a day for children between nine and twelve years of age. In severely refractory older children, imipramine could cautiously be increased to 100 mg. twice a day.

The duration of treatment should be approximately six weeks if good results are obtained. The primary target symptom is the child's anxiety. School attendance and performance are undoubtedly important, but still secondary in significance. Although Gittelman-Klein and Klein (1973) report treating some children for more than six months, we suggest discontinuing the medication if there is no response after three months or reducing medication to a much lower maintenance dose (approximately one-half of the maximum) if there has been some improvement.

The only significant side effect as compared with placebo reported by Gittelman-Klein and Klein (1973) was dry mouth. Other frequently reported side effects included drowsiness, dizziness, constipation, nausea, indigestion, anorexia, increased appetite, and mild tremor and sweating. Other side effects, such as hypotension and rarely, hypertension, cardiac conduction abnormalities, and liver and blood toxicities, have been reported frequently enough in adults that the physician must observe carefully for these side effects.

The following procedure is recommended for monitoring of side effects or toxicity: Prior to initiating treatment, the usual complete history including drug sensitivity reactions should be elicited and a thorough physical examination performed. Routine chest X ray and EKG should be taken, and if any conduction abnormalities, congenital defects or abnormalities of the heart are noted, imipramine treatment should not be initiated. CBC and liver profile should be normal, or imipramine treatment should not be started. Careful blood-pressure evaluation with lying and immediate standing readings should be done to document any preexisting postural hypotension or hypertension. The patient should be seen one week after starting treatment, prior to the second increase in dosage or earlier if any symptoms are reported. At the first follow-up examination, careful blood-pressure readings again should be obtained and pulse regularity assessed carefully. If any deviation from normal is found, a repeat EKG should be performed. If no other symptoms or signs of toxicity are obtained, the patient then should be seen at weekly intervals. Once satisfactory results have been obtained, the imipramine should be tapered over a one-week period rather than abruptly withdrawn (Greenberg and Roth, 1966). Initially the tapering can be rather rapid, but there should be at least a three- or four-day terminal period with the patient on minimal doses of approximately 25 mg./day in order to avoid the malaise and general discomfort that accompanies abrupt termination of imipramine. The patient and the parents should be seen at monthly intervals until completion of the school term to be certain that the child's anxiety has been treated adequately.

Monoamine oxidase inhibitors have held a controversial place in psychopharmacological treatment. Dramatic success was reported from England (Frommer, 1967, 1968) with a combination of MAO inhibitor and minor tranquilizer in treatment of refractory school phobias. Gittelman-Klein (1975) also reported the use of an MAO inhibitor in five cases refractory to imipramine, but only one patient improved. Since the MAO inhibitors are so toxic and not known to be superior to imipramine, we feel that their use is contraindicated in cases of school refusal except in extremely unusual circumstances.

The mode of action of imipramine in this illness is not any better understood than the etiology and psychopathology of school phobias. Various authors feel that the medication acts by modifying an underlying depression (Frommer, 1967, 1968) or a primary separation anxiety (Gittelman-Klein and Klein, 1973). It may in fact be that there are different subtypes of school phobias and that school phobia represents an end result of complex interaction of many factors. Hope-

fully, as suggested by Gittelman-Klein (1975), the advent of psychopharmacological treatment for severe, refractory cases will contribute to a better understanding of this disorder. Certainly, psychopharmacology is a very important
part of the psychiatrist's armamentarium in the treatment of the school phobias.

ANOREXIA NERVOSA

The final section of this chapter deals with anorexia nervosa. It is a short section
since the use of psychoactive medications, particularly the phenothiazines, has
received little or no systematic study. Although the efficacy of these medications
in the treatment of anorexia nervosa is unknown, clinicians do frequently prescribe them as an adjunctive treatment.

Anorexia nervosa generally is considered to involve "self-inflicted starvation" (Bruch, 1966) or "psychogenic malnutrition" (Branch and Bliss, 1967).
Beyond a basic agreement that patients with weight loss caused by primary physical pathology are excluded, there is considerable disagreement among various
authors about the criteria for diagnosis of anorexia nervosa. Bliss and Branch
(1960) add only the criterion of a minimum of twenty-five pounds weight loss
and included patients with schizophrenia, depression, and hysteria. However,
there is a clear trend toward the use of more selective criteria to differentiate the
specific entity, anorexia nervosa, in keeping with the first descriptions of this
syndrome by Gull and Laseque in the 1870s. Dally and Sargant (1960) require
five criteria: 1. refusal to eat whether or not accompanied by anorexia; 2. a
minimum weight loss of 10 percent of the permorbid body weight; 3. amenorrhea
of at least three months' duration or if menstruation has not begun, a minimum
age of sixteen years; 4. no evidence of schizophrenia, severe depression, or
organic disease; and 5. a maximum age at onset of thirty-five years. However, by
definition, they exclude male patients. Bruch (1966, 1973) includes female and
male patients, but otherwise suggests perhaps the most restrictive criteria for her
general definition of "self-inflicted starvation without recognizable organic disease and in the midst of ample food." She quite correctly excludes all "hunger
strikes" in the tradition of Gandhi, religious fasts, and all "instances of undernu-
trition secondary to a well defined psychiatric illness." Further, she subdivides
the remaining group of anorexia nervosa patients into two subtypes which require
careful evaluation and psychodynamic assessment. The first subgroup, "atypical
anorexia nervosa," involves patients with "an eating function which was used in
various symbolic ways . . . the loss of weight was incidental to some other
problem, and it was often complained of or valued only secondarily for its course

of effect . . . cases of refusal to eat in the service of neurotic or schizophrenic conflicts.'' The second subgroup, ''true anorexia nervosa,'' is characterized by three diagnostic features: the body-image disturbance of delusional proportions; disturbance in the accuracy of perception of bodily states including failure to recognize the signs of nutritional needs and paradoxic overactivity of the patients; and pervading sense of ineffectiveness representing a defect in personality development. Crisp (1974) suggests the terms ''primary anorexia nervosa or adolescent weight phobia,'' and implies, in succinct British fashion, that the following doctor-patient interchange is diagnostic. Doctor's question: If you could eat like other people and yet not gain any weight, would you do so? Patient's answer: Yes.

There does seem to be a clear consensus that anorexia nervosa is predominantly an illness of female patients. The proportions range widely, however, from 20:1 to 5:1 with an apparent compromise in the range of 10:1 females over males.

The actual incidence and prevalence are unknown although the diagnosis appears to be made with increasing frequency. Crisp (1974) suggests that it ''probably exists in severe form in roughly one in every 150 school girls aged 16–18 years.'' Although the usual age of onset is not agreed upon, some authors report prepubertal cases as well as cases with an onset in the fifties. Usually, however, the onset is during adolescence (Bruch, 1966; Crisp, 1974) at or after puberty and before age eighteen. Some cases with an apparent onset after age eighteen years may have begun earlier with a relatively mild dieting ritual.

Many clinical features are generally recognized to have diagnostic importance, but are not necessarily present in each case. The overactivity of these patients is a well-recognized symptom. A striking lack of concern by these patients for their weight loss and cachexia commonly is reported, and they often see no need for any treatment whatsoever. Primary or secondary amenorrhea is a frequent finding. Secondary sexual characteristics and pubic hair appear to be relatively well preserved. Endocrine studies are generally within normal limits with the exception of the gonadotropic hormones. These patients frequently report marked anxiety, uneasiness, or fear within a few minutes to an hour prior to mealtime. There are a variety of bizarre behaviors included among the ''food rituals.'' These patients frequently develop an intense interest in food and gourmet cooking, and prepare elaborate meals for other family members, but not themselves. They may indulge in ''food binges'' or bulimia which usually are followed very rapidly by spontaneous or induced vomiting and excessive use of laxatives and enemas. Since these patients often are rather chubby prior to puberty, initial dieting efforts appear normal; thus, there is a delay in seeking medical attention. These patients often are deceptive about their weight and add weights to their pockets or drink considerable water prior to being weighed. They may hide their food in dresser drawers, corners of closets, toys, and other inappropriate places with petulant and immature reactions when confronted.

The natural course of the illness is not well known. Crisp (1974) suggests that there are two general patterns. The first group with early spontaneous remission, sometimes followed by mild obesity, regularly exacerbate with frequent medical crises. The prognosis is relatively poor with 6 to 10 percent mortality in patients with this form of the disease for ten years or more. Death is usually from inanition or actual suicide. Crisp describes the second group as remaining chronically ill and cachectic appearing but somehow avoiding medical crisis. They live "mainly as thin, eccentric spinsters, often obviously involved in bizarre dietary practices." However, by the fifth and sixth decade of life they frequently recover.

There is no attempt in this section to deal with the acute medical management of the seriously malnourished patient. Patients are seen with serious metabolic changes and marked electrolyte abnormalities (particularly elevated serum potassium). These situations are life threatening and must be treated in a medical intensive-care unit. Upon initial improvement in nourishment, serious medical complications such as edema, congestive heart failure, and cardiac arrhythmias can occur. However, considerable debate continues (Moldofsky and Garfinkel, 1974) about the value of tube and intravenous feedings. There is some evidence that the risks of pulmonary aspiration, infection, and death from tube feedings and of metabolic disturbances with intravenous fluids may carry a greater risk than the actual starvation itself. Also, anesthesia for ECT in these severe cases carries a high risk. Newer techniques of intravenous hyperalimentation utilizing amino acid precursors appear promising.

Psychotherapeutic interventions with these patients have tended to follow the prevailing psychodynamic formulation for the illness. Earlier analytic formulations involving fears of oral impregnation and pregnancy fantasies (Waller, Kaufman, and Deutsch, 1940) largely have been discarded (Galdston, 1974). More recent analytic formulations involving drive disturbances and oral ambivalence (Thomae, 1961) do not appear to have rendered analysis of any value in this illness (Bruch, 1966). Family psychopathology certainly is found with great frequency but may be secondary to the anorexia nervosa. Many authors do recommend family therapy as part of the total management of this illness (Liebman, Minuchin, and Baker, 1974; Crisp, 1974). Recent psychodynamic formulations and treatment (Bruch, 1966, 1973) emphasized the disturbances in body-image concept, perception of bodily states of nutrition and activity, and a sense of ineffectiveness; she recommends a more direct psychotherapeutic approach.

Behavioral therapies have become increasingly popular and the results, at least short-term, are very encouraging. A typical treatment plan as proposed by

Stunkard (1972) involves picking appropriate contingencies that are attractive enough to the patient to result in a daily weight gain. Contingencies such as physical exercise and activity frequently are negotiated for weight gains of one-half pound each day.

Psychopharmacological treatment has played a definite role in the treatment of anorexia nervosa since 1960 when Dally and Sargant (1966) described much greater short-term success when chlorpromazine was used in addition to the standard bed-rest and insulin treatments. The use of phenothiazines, based on fortuitous clinical observations, has come to be a nearly standard part of the overall management of anorexia nervosa, even in the face of a serious lack of any well-controlled or blind studies. As described by Dally and Sargant (1966), rather large doses of chlorpromazine are used, starting at approximately 300 mg./day and increasing slowly to as high as 1,600 mg./day. More conservatively, Crisp (1965) recommended an average dose of chlorpromazine of about 400 mg./day. Probably any of the phenothiazines or haloperidol would have a similar success, but comparative studies are inadequate. The mechanism of action is not known.

Specific pharmacological treatment for weight gain has been unsuccessful in anorexia nervosa. The original enthusiasm for the histamine and serotonin antagonist, periactin, which was found to induce significant weight gain in asthmatic children, has faded (Anderson, 1974). Similarly, treatment with various anabolic steroids generally has been unsuccessful (Anderson, 1974).

None of the above treatment modalities has proved to be significantly effective in the long-term management of these patients. Even with behavior therapy, phenothiazine treatment and psychotherapy in several studies (summarized in Moldofsky and Garfinkel, 1974) have a recurrence of symptoms in approximately 25–50 percent of patients regardless of treatment.

SUMMARY *

These special syndromes of enuresis, Gilles de la Tourette's syndrome, school phobia, and anorexia nervosa represent a heterogeneous grouping whose only relationship is that each lends itself to fairly precise definition.

Enuresis and school phobia are relatively common, while anorexia and the tic syndrome are less frequent in incidence. Many cases of enuresis and probably all valid cases of the Gilles de la Tourette syndrome are related to neurophysiological and neurotransmittor factors respectively; such factors have not been iden-

* Editor's summary.

tified or seriously suggested by the available data either in school-phobia or "typical" anorexia nervosa cases.

Concomitantly, drug therapy is most specific for the Gilles de la Tourette syndrome, wherein administration of haloperidol in accurately diagnosed cases can result in a remission rate of up to 90 percent, making it one of the most specific treatments available in the field of psychopharmacology. Use of the tricyclic antidepressants, most commonly imipramine, in the treatment of enuresis has far less specificity. Nevertheless it can be an effective treatment in a responder population, and differential treatment results beyond the placebo effect can be related to the pharmacological properties of the drugs used.

Of primary importance in the Gilles de la Tourette syndrome is accuracy in diagnosis—to avoid positive errors, because haloperidol is a potent drug in the dosage ranges often required for effective results in this condition and, of utmost importance, to avoid negative errors, because of the above-mentioned specificity and effectiveness of this treatment.

For cases of enuresis a careful examination for physical causes and a comprehensive evaluation of the total personality and family context is most important. Here medication with imipramine is adjunctive, rarely primary, and often unnecessary when other modalities are appropriately used. Successful management in any event will require the cooperative involvement of the family and the child. Where reeducative, supportive, and, when indicated, psychotherapeutic measures are insufficient, imipramine is more likely to be effective with secondary enuretics without other significant neurotic symptoms or other associated behavioral problems.

School refusal is a behavioral constellation specifically described over thirty years ago (as "school phobia"), and most commonly accepted as related to the dynamics of undue separation anxiety. Only in the past few years has medication been advocated on the basis of results obtained from methodologically sound studies. In these studies (Gittleman-Klein, 1975; Gittleman-Klein and Klein, 1973) the tricyclic antidepressant imipramine, in relatively high doses for the pediatric age group, proved significantly superior to placebo in alleviating the anxiety and facilitating return to school. Imipramine at high-dosage levels must be used with clinical caution and awareness of the potential for cardiac arrhythmia as a side effect, requiring a decision in each case on the basis of the benefit/risk ratio. In selected cases, however, the use of imipramine may represent a valuable addition to the traditional approaches.

Although phenothiazines are not uncommonly used in the treatment of anorexia nervosa, there are no well-controlled studies or systematic data supporting its use. As an adjunct to a variety of other approaches (individual and family therapy, behavior modification) the use of the phenothiazines remains an individualized clinical decision.

210   LAWRENCE M. GREENBERG & JAMES H. STEPHANS

It may be reemphasized that in these special syndromes there is a great diversity and no substitute for experienced and sophisticated clinical judgment for both evaluation and accurate diagnosis on the one hand, and comprehensive treatment planning on the other.

References

Abuzzahab, F. (1976), Personal communication.
Anderson, J. (1974), Drugs and appetite. *The Practitioner, 212,* 536–544.
Arnold, S. J., and Ginsburg, A. (1973), Enuresis: Incidence and pertinence of genitourinary disease in healthy enuretic children. *Urology,* 1973, *11,* 437–443.
Berg, I., Marks, I., McGuire, R., and Lipsedge, M. (1974), School phobia and agoraphobia. *Psych. Med., 4,* 428–434.
Berger, H. G. (1974), Somatic pain and school avoidance. *Clin. Ped., 13,* 819–826.
Blackwell, B., and Currah, J. (1973), The psychopharmacology of nocturnal enuresis. In I. Kolvin, R. C. MacKeith, and S. R. Meadow (Eds.), *Bladder control and enuresis.* Philadelphia: J. B. Lippincott, Co., pp. 231–257.
Bliss, E. L., and Branch, C. H. (1960), *Anorexia nervosa.* New York: Hoeber.
Branch, C. H., and Bliss, E. L. (1967), Anorexia nervosa. In A. M. Freedman, and H. I. Kaplan (Eds.), *Comprehensive textbook of psychiatry.* Baltimore: Williams and Wilkins, pp. 1062–1063.
Bruch, H. (1966), Anorexia nervosa and its differential diagnosis. *J. Nerv. and Ment. Dis., 141,* 555–566.
Bruch, H. (1973), *Eating disorders: Obesity, anorexia nervosa and the person within.* New York: Basic Books.
Brunn, R. D., and Shapiro, A. K. (1972), Differential diagnosis of Gilles de la Tourette's Syndrome. *J. Nerv. and Ment. Dis., 154,* 328–334.
Chapel, J. L. (1970), Latah, myriachit, and jumpers revisited. *N. Y. St. J. Med., 70,* 2201–2204.
Corbett, J. A., Mathews, A. M., Connel, P. H., and Shapiro, D. A. (1969), Tics and Gilles de la Tourette's syndrome: A follow-up study and critical review. *Brit. J. Psychiat., 115,* 1229–1241.
Corbin, K. B. (1970), Common neurophysiologic factors reported in literature. *N. Y. St. J. Med., 70,* 2193–2200.
Crisp, A. H. (1965), Clinical and therapeutic aspects of anorexia nervosa—a study of thirty cases. *J. Psychosom. Res., 9,* 67–68.
Crisp, A. H. (1974), Primary anorexia nervosa or adolescent weight phobia. *The Practitioner, 212,* 525–535.
Dally, P. J., and Sargant, W. (1960), A new treatment of anorexia nervosa. *Brit. Med. J., 1,* 1770–1772.
Dally, P. J., and Sargant, W. (1966), Treatment and outcome of anorexia nervosa. *Brit. Med. J., 2,* 793–795.
Dische, S. (1973), Treatment of enuresis with an enuresis alarm. In I. Kolvin, R. C. MacKeith, and S. R. Meadows (Eds.), *Bladder control and enuresis.* Clinics in Developmental Medicine Nos. 48/49. Philadelphia: Lippincott Co..
Eisenberg, L. (1958), School phobia: A study in the communication of anxiety. *Am. J. Psychiat., 114,* 712–718.
Fisher, G. W., Murray, F., Walley, M. R., and Kiloh, L. G. (1963), A controlled trial of imipramine in the treatment of nocturnal enuresis in mentally subnormal patients. *Am. J. Ment. Def., 67,* 536.
Forsythe, W. I., and Merit, J. D. (1969), A controlled trial of imipramine ('Tofranil') and nortriptyline ('Allegron') in the treatment of enuresis. *Brit. J. Clin. Prac., 23,* 210–215.
Forsythe, W. I., and Redmond, A. (1974), Enuresis and spontaneous cure rate: Study of 1129 enuretics. *Arch. Dis. Ch., 49,* 259–263.
Friel, P. B. (1973), Familial incidence of Gilles de la Tourette's Disease, with observations on aetiology and treatment. *Brit. J. Psychiat., 122,* 655–658.

Frommer, E. A. (1967), Treatment of childhood depression with antidepressant drug. *Brit. J. Med.,* *1,* 729–732.

Frommer, E. A. Depressive illness in childhood (1968), In A. Coppen, and A. Walk (Eds.), *Recent developments in affective disorders. Brit. J. Psychiat.,* Special Publ. No. 2, pp. 117–136.

Galdston, R. (1974), Mind over matter: Observations on 50 patients hospitalized with anorexia nervosa. *J. Am. Acad. Ch. Psychiat., 13,* 246–265.

Gittleman-Klein, R. (1975), Pharmacotherapy and management of pathological separation anxiety. *Int. J. Ment. Health, 4,* 255–271.

Gittelman-Klein, R., and Klein, D. (1973), School phobia: Diagnostic considerations in the light of imipramine effects. *J. Nerv. & Ment. Dis., 156,* 199–215.

Glicklich, L. B. (1951), An historical account of enuresis. *Pediatrics, 8,* 859–876.

Gold, T. L., Kline, N. S., and Winick, L. (1969), Drug evaluation of private practice: A comparison of drug response in patients under 21 years of age. *Psychosomatics, 10,* 39–42.

Greenberg, L. M., and Roth, S. (1966), Differential effects of abrupt versus gradual withdrawal of chlorpromazine in hospitalized, schizophrenic patients. *Am. J. Psychiat., 123,* 221–225.

Greenberg, L. M., and Yellin, A. M. (1975), Blood pressure and pulse changes in hyperactive children treated with imipramine and methylphenidate. *Am. J. Psychiat., 132,* 1325–1326.

Hersov, L. A. (1960), Persistent non-attendance at school. *J. Ch. Psych. & Psychiat., 1,* 130–136.

Johnson, A. M., Falstein, E. I., Szurek, S. A., and Svendsen, M. (1941), School phobia. *Am. J. Orthopsychiat., 11,* 702–711.

Kanner, L. (1957), *Child psychiatry.* Springfield: Charles C. Thomas.

Kellmer Pringle, M. L., Butler, N. R., and Davie, R. (1967), Tics in *11,000 seven years olds.* London: National Bureau for Cooperation in Child Care, p. 185.

Kennedy, W. A. (1965), School phobia: Rapid treatment of fifty cases. *J. Ab. Psych.,* 1965, *70,* 285–289.

Kessler, J. W. (1972), Neurosis in childhood. In B. B. Wolman (Ed.), *Manual of child psychopathology.* New York: McGraw-Hill, pp. 387–435.

Kolvin, I., Garside, R. F., Taunch, J., Currah, J., and McNay, R. A. (1973), Feature clustering and prediction of improvement in nocturnal enuresis. In I. Kolvin, R. C. MacKeith, and S. R. Meadow (Eds.), *Bladder control and enuresis.* Philadelphia: J. B. Lippincott, pp. 258–284.

Lake, B. (1968), Controlled trial of nortriptyline in childhood enuresis. *Med. J. of Australia, 2,* 582–585.

Lansky, S., Lowman, J. T., Vats, T., and Gyulay, J-E (1975), School phobia in children with malignant neoplasms. *Am. J. Dis. Ch.,* 1975, *129,* 42–46.

Liebman, R., Minuchin, S., and Baker, L. (1974), An integrated treatment program for anorexia nervosa. *Am. J. Psychiat., 131,* 432–436.

Lucas, A. R. (1967), Gilles de la Tourette's disease in children: Treatment with haloperidol. *Am. J. Psychiat., 124,* 147–149.

Lucas, A. R. (1970), Gilles de la Tourette's disease: An overview. *N.Y. State J. Med., 70,* 2197–2200.

Lucas, A. R., Kauffman, P. E., and Morris, E. M. (1967), Gilles de la Tourette's disease: A clinical study of fifteen cases. *J. Am. Acad. Ch. Psychiat., 6,* 700–722.

MacLean, R. E. G. (1960), Imipramine hydrochloride (Tofranil) and enuresis. *Am. J. Psychiat., 117,* 551.

Mahler, M. R. L. (1943), A psychosomatic study of maladiedtics. *Psychiatric Quarterly, 17,* 579.

Mahler, M. S., Luke, J. A., and Daltroff, W. (1945), Clinical and follow-up study of the tic syndrome in children. *Am. J. Orthopsychiat., 15,* 631–647.

Malmquist, C. P. (1965), School phobia: A problem in family neurosis. *J. Ch. Psychiatry, 4,* 293–319.

Martin, G. I., and Zaug, P. J. (1975), Electrocardiographic monitoring of enuretic children receiving therapeutic doses of imipramine. *Am. J. Psychiat., 132,* 540–542.

McKendry, J. B. J., and Stewart, D. A. (1974), Enuresis. *Ped. Clin. N. Am., 24,* 1019–1027.

McLellan, F. C. (1939), *The Neurogenic Bladder.* Springfield: Charles C. Thomas.

Meadow, R. (1973), Practical aspects of the management of nocturnal enuresis. In I. Kolvin, R. C. MacKeith, and S. R. Meadow (Eds.), *Bladder control and enuresis.* Philadelphia: J. B. Lippincott, Co., pp. 181–188.

Meadow, R. (1974), Drugs for bed-wetting. *Arch. Dis. Ch., 49,* 257–258.

Miller, L. C., Hampe, E., Barrett, C. L., and Noble, H. (1971), Children's deviant behavior within the general population. *J. of Consult. & Clin. Psych., 37,* 16–22.

Milner, G., & Hills, N. F. (1968), A double-blind assessment of antidepressants in the treatment of 212 enuretic patients. *Med. J. of Australia, 1,*943–947.

Mitchell, S., and Shepherd, M. (1967), The child who dislikes going to school. *Brit. J. of Ed. Psych., 37,*32–40.

Moldofsky, H., and Garfinkel, P. E. (1974), Problems of treatment of anorexia nervosa. *Can. Psychiatr. Assn. J., 19,*169–175.

Oppel, W. C., Harper, P. A., and Rider, R. V. (1968), The age of attaining bladder control. *Pediatrics, 42,*614–641.

Perel, J. (1975), Recent advances in psychopharmacology. Presented at the American Academy of Child Psychiatry meeting, St. Louis, Missouri, October 20, 1976.

Petersen, K. E., Andersen, O. O., and Hansen, T. (1974), Mode of action and relative value of imipramine and similar drugs in the treatment of nocturnal enuresis. *Eur. J. Clin. Pharm., 7,*187–194.

Poussaint, A. F., and Ditman, K. S. (1965), A controlled study of imipramine (Tofranil) in the treatment of childhood enuresis. *J. Ped., 67,*283–290.

Ritvo, E. R., Ornitz, E. M., LaFranchi, S., and Walter, R. D. (1967), Effects of imipramine on the sleep-dream cycle: An EEG study in boys. *Electroencephalograph and Clin. Neurophys., 22,*465.

Ritvo, E. R., Ornitz, E. M., Gottlieb, R., Poussaint, A. F., Maron, B. J., Ditman, K. S., and Blinn, K. A. (1969), Arousal and nonarousal enuretic events. *Am. J. Psychiat., 126,*77–84.

Rodriguez, A., Rodriguez, M., and Eisenberg, L. (1959), The outcome of school phobia: A follow-up study based on 41 cases. *Am. J. Psychiat., 116,*540–544.

Sanders, D. G. (1973), Familial occurrence of Gilles de la Tourette syndrome. *Arch. Gen. Psychiat., 28,* 326–328.

Saraf, K. R., Klein, D. F., Gittelman-Klein, R., and Groff, S. (1974), Imipramine side effects in children. *Psychopharmacologia* (Berlin), 37, 265.

Shaffer, D. (1973), The association between enuresis and emotional disorders: Review of literature. In I. Kolvin, R. C. MacKeith, and S. R. Meadow (Eds.), *Bladder control and enuresis.* Philadelphia: J. B. Lippincott, pp. 118–136.

Shaffer, D., Costello, A. J., and Hill, I. D. (1968), Control of enuresis with imipramine. *Arch. Dis. Ch., 43,*665–671.

Shapiro, A. K. (1970), Symposium on Gilles de la Tourette syndrome. *N. Y. St. J. Med., 70,*2193–2214.

Shapiro, A., Shapiro, E., and Wayne, H. (1972a), Birth, developmental, and family histories and demographic information in Tourette's syndrome. *J. Nerv. & Ment. Dis., 155,*335–344.

Shapiro, A. K., Shapiro, E., Wayne, H., and Clarkin, J. (1972b), The psychopathology of Gilles de la Tourette's syndrome. *Am. J. Psychiat., 129,*427–434.

Shapiro, A. K., Shapiro, E., and Wayne, H. L. (1973a), The symptomatology and diagnosis of Gilles de la Tourette's syndrome. *J. Am. Acad. Ch. Psychiat., 12,*702–723.

Shapiro, A. K., Shapiro, E., Wayne, H., and Clarkin, J. (1973b), Organic factors in Gilles de la Tourette's Syndrome. *Brit. J. Psychiat., 122,*659–664.

Shapiro, A. K., Shapiro, E., Wayne, H., Clarkin, J., and Brunn, R. D. (1973c), Tourette's Syndrome: Summary of data on 34 patients. *Psychosom. Med., 34,*419–435.

Skynner, A. C. R. (1974), School phobia, a reappraisal, *Brit. J. Med. Psych., 47,*1–16.

Sperling, M. (1967), School phobias: Classification, dynamics and treatment. *Psychoanal. Study of the Child, 22,*375.

Stunkard, A. (1972), New therapies for the eating disorders. *Arch. Gen. Psychiat., 26,*391–398.

Thomae, H. (1961), *Anorexia nervosa,* Bern-Stuttgart: Huber-Klett.

Torup, E. (1962), A follow-up study of children with tics. *Acta. Paediat., 51,*261–268.

Troup, C. W., and Hodgson, N. B. (1971), Nocturnal functional bladder capacity in enuretic children. *Ped. Urol., 105,*129–132.

Turner, R. K. (1973), Conditioning treatment of nocturnal enuresis: Present status. In I. Kolvin, R. C. MacKeith, & S. R. Meadow (Eds.), *Bladder control and enuresis.* Philadelphia: J. B. Lippincott, pp. 195–210.

Tyrer, P., and Tyrer, S. (1974), School refusal, truancy, and adult neurotic illness. *Psych. Med., 4,*416–421.

Waller, J. V., Kaufman, and Deutsch, F. (1940), Anorexia nervosa: A psychosomatic entity. *Psychosom. Med., 2,* 3–16.

Warren, W. (1965), A study of adolescent psychiatric inpatients and the outcome six or more years later: 2. The follow-up study. *J. Ch. Psych. & Psychiat., 6,* 141–160.

Woodrow, K. M. (1974), Gilles de la Tourette's Disease: A review. *Am. J. Psychiat., 131,* 1000–1003.

Yodfat, Y. (1966), Treatment of enuresis. *Lancet, 1,* 368.

Part III

CONCLUSION AND PROSPECT

Chapter Ten

SUMMARY

Jerry M. Wiener, M.D.

If taken from its first specific origins in the 1930s, the field of childhood psychopharmacology per se is not young. If viewed, however, by criteria for scientific maturity, it is still early in its development, but past its infancy and growing rapidly. A bit like the active toddler, the field is going in many different directions at once, still a bit diffuse and unfocussed, not yet completely steady on its underpinnings, and with a lot of basic growth yet to be realized; but also very robust, its basic equipment (methodology) acquired and intact, steadily learning new information, gaining balance, and establishing a clear identity in the family of therapies.

Like its sibling clinical discipline of child psychiatry, childhood and adolescent psychopharmacology has followed behind and often been dependent upon the discoveries and advances in adult psychopharmacology. Medications that were effective (or thought to be so) for the treatment of adult psychopathology have then been prescribed for the child, as homunculus, for conditions with similar symptomatology, or in many cases for conditions with dissimilar symptomatology, but with the same label as the adult illness (e.g., schizophrenia). The major exception to this repeated sequence of events was the use of stimulant drugs for the treatment of hyperactivity.

The field of childhood psychopharmacology has developed much as child psychiatry itself, at first located in community child-guidance clinics and in freestanding mental institutions which were separated from the mainstream of medical practice and also from the influence of academic medicine and even academic psychiatry; and then moving progressively back into practice and training in academic university programs and hospital-affiliated services. Likewise, research in drug treatment of children has moved from noncontrolled studies with poorly defined heterogeneous populations to an increasingly more self-critical and rigorous methodology. This now includes all the accepted criteria for obtaining reliable and valid data, and an increasingly sophisticated consideration of the special problems, methodological and ethical, of drug research and drug treatment in an immature, constantly changing, and developing subject population.

This book has intended to be a comprehensive review of the evolving state of both the art and the science of childhood and adolescent psychopharmacology. Its aim is at both a breadth and depth that will make it useful to clinicians at varying levels of specialization, including the family practitioner, pediatrician, internist dealing with adolescents, the general and the child psychiatrist, allied health and mental health professionals, and to the psychodynamic as well as to the more biologically oriented clinician. While this is a widely thrown net, the field itself is still of a size that can be comprehensively encompassed in a single volume. Its contents can be turned to as a source for classification and pharmacology, guidelines for methods of evaluation and implementation of drug studies or clinical trials, as a theoretical consideration of drug interaction with the developmental process, for comprehensive presentations of both the clinical syndromes and clinical use of drugs in their treatment, and for an extensive reference bibliography.

At its core, however, the book provides information to clinicians treating childhood and adolescent psychopathology, covering the indications, contraindications, valid expectations, recommended approaches, and side effects of psychoactive drugs. From this perspective several themes are emphasized throughout the various chapters:

1. Drug therapy is almost always to be considered adjunctive and not the only or even the primary treatment.

2. Only in a few defined syndromes or diagnoses (Gilles de la Tourette syndrome, childhood psychosis, primary enuresis) should drug therapy be an initial rather than a later or concomitant therapeutic approach.

3. The decision to use drugs should in all cases be preceded by a proper history, family, and psychosocial evaluation, direct examination of the child (including his mental status), psychological evaluation, and a determination of his neurological status.

4. Drug therapy should be part of a formulated treatment plan with specific, defined goals, including careful follow-up and monitoring for side effects.

5. The practitioner should be familiar with one drug out of each class or group, and begin drug treatment with the minimum therapeutic dose for that drug and increase the dose until satisfactory clinical benefit or interfering side effects occur. Drug-free trials should then be a standard part of almost every drug treatment in a child, with an aim toward a minimum maintenance dose and the earliest point at which drug therapy can be discontinued. Much remains unknown

about the effects of psychoactive agents on the developmental process itself and about the possible long-term adverse effects of drugs.

6. The practitioner should not set aside or overlook, in favor of drug therapy, the other time-tested therapeutic interventions indicated for either the primary consequences or the secondary effects of the condition under treatment. These interventions include the various psychotherapeutic approaches—individual, group, family, couples—as well as environmental, psychosocial, and psycho-educational considerations.

Having emphasized these precautions, it is also appropriate to repeat a quotation from an earlier chapter: ". . . it is an error of equal magnitude [to the inappropriate or excessive use of drugs] to deny a patient an agent which can help relieve his symptoms and hasten his recovery." (Eisenberg and Conners, 1971; quoted by Patterson and Pruitt, ch. seven.) Although the overall tone of this book is intentionally and, for the current state of the field, appropriately conservative, it is certainly not nihilistic or negative in its recommendations and guidelines for specific drug therapy.

More important, the field is expanding and growing in a now more systematic and reliable fashion, increasingly related to specific developmental considerations, and it is on the threshold of correlations between clinical studies and advancing knowledge about biological mechanisms in psychopathology.

It is worthwhile identifying those issues and trends in the field that represent present areas of activity and hold promise for and point to the future:

1. There is an increasing attention to the importance of diagnosis per se and to diagnostic specificity in childhood and adolescent disorders. The field has passed through, and is now emerging from, the nonmedical or antimedical attitudes and models which came into vogue with the community mental health center movement. Paradoxically, in many community mental health centers, the psychiatrist and child psychiatrist were and still are regarded as necessary only for the prescription of medication, while diagnosis and careful observation of results were devalued as irrelevant intrusions of the medical model, and perhaps at best pejorative and useless labeling. An understandable, but nonetheless ultimately self-defeating antagonism to any suggestion of investigation or research also came to be an associated aspect of this attitude.

In all fairness, this question of diagnosis has been debated within psychiatry itself, generating more heat than light, but now seems to occur more at the periphery rather than at the center of psychiatric concern.

In childhood disorders, where great diagnostic disarray has been more a rule than an exception, advances in diagnostic precision have been often intertwined with and stimulated by opportunities to introduce medication as part of treatment.

Infantile autism, childhood schizophrenia, the minimal brain dysfunction syndrome, anorexia nervosa, and depression are examples of diagnostic categories for which increasingly precise and descriptive criteria are being defined. The trend will undoubtedly continue and reflect, as well as allow, more meaningful integrations of biological, psychodynamic, and psychosocial sources of information for understanding etiology, pathology, treatment, and prognosis, all of which ideally should be communicated in a diagnostic label.

2. Advances in our understanding of brain activity at the neurophysiological, biochemical, neuroendocrine, and neuropsychological levels of investigation is literally an exploding field, making a major impact on child psychiatry in the past few years. One major stimulus has been the need to understand the clues and leads provided by the effects on behavior and symptoms of the phenothiazine and antidepressant drugs introduced during the 1950s and 1960s. Another lead has come from the observed similarity in adults between the effects of psychotomimetic drugs and abuse of stimulant medication to the symptoms of schizophrenia. Further support for biochemical investigations has come from the demonstration of a genetic component in the transmission of schizophrenia. In childhood disorders investigative activity is concentrated on the neurophysiology, biochemistry and genetics of childhood autism, the broader syndrome of childhood schizophrenia, minimal brain dysfunction and associated learning disability syndromes, and childhood depression. These investigations and the effect of medication reported in such diverse syndromes or symptoms as enuresis, school phobia, and the Gilles de la Tourette syndrome raise intriguing questions and present the opportunity for fresh hypotheses about the interaction of endogenous and experiential factors not only for these conditions, but with application to other disorders and normal development as well.

3. Collaboration between the behavioral, clinical, and biological sciences is increasingly fostered and required for sufficient conceptualizations of both normal and deviant developmental and behavioral outcomes. It seems clear as things now stand, that no one perspective (biochemical, genetic, psychoanalytic, developmental, etc.) is alone sufficient to address either etiology or treatment. It also seems clear that for the near future the major advances in our understanding will come from discoveries in biological psychiatry as understood and applied by sophisticated clinicians.

4. In psychopharmacology we can expect a period of solid progress and achievement in better understanding:

a.   mechanism and site of action
b.   the pharmacokinetics and dispositional characteristics of the drugs we use
c.   the relationship between drug effect and the pathophysiology of the illness
d.   the conditions that influence response (e.g., developmental, psychological, familial) and identify responders from nonresponders

e. the longer-term effect of drugs on clinical course, prognosis, and on the developmental process itself

We are entering a period in which a rational psychopharmacology will increasingly be available for childhood and adolescent disorders. It is an exciting prospect, both for primary treatment where justified, and as an adjunctive facilitator for other more traditional educative and psychotherapeutic approaches. Both for a better understanding of the clinical syndromes and for specific guidelines to drug treatment, the clinician will be amply guided by the information provided in this book. Beyond that, practitioners and students at all levels may be comprehensively informed by both the first and second sections on the breadth of considerations applicable to the decision to introduce psychoactive medication in the treatment of children and adolescents.

The contributors to this book have provided a detailed description of where we have come from, where we are now, and where we need to go.

INDEX